Underground Clinical Vignettes

Pathophysiology II: GI, Neurology,
Rheumatology, Endocrinology

FIFTH EDITION

Underground Clinical Vignettes

Pathophysiology II: GI, Neurology, Rheumatology, Endocrinology

FIFTH EDITION

Todd A. Swanson, M.D., Ph.D.
Resident in Radiation Oncology
William Beaumont Hospital
Royal Oak, Michigan

Sandra I. Kim, M.D., Ph.D.
Resident in Internal Medicine
Beth Israel Deaconess Medical Center
Harvard Medical School
Boston, Massachusetts

Olga E. Flomin, M.D.
Resident in Obstetrics and Gynecology
William Beaumont Hospital
Royal Oak, Michigan

Wolters Kluwer | Lippincott Williams & Wilkins
Health
Philadelphia · Baltimore · New York · London
Buenos Aires · Hong Kong · Sydney · Tokyo

Acquisitions editor: Nancy Anastasi Duffy
Developmental editor: Kathleen H. Scogna
Managing Editor: Nancy Hoffmann
Marketing manager: Jennifer Kuklinski
Associate Production Manager: Kevin Johnson
Creative Director: Doug Smock
Compositor: International Typesetting and Composition
Printer: R.R. Donnelley & Son's—Crawfordsville

Printed in the United States of America

First Edition, 2001 Blackwell Publishing Inc.
Second Edition, 2003 Blackwell Publishing Inc.
Third Edition, 2005 Blackwell Publishing Inc.
Fourth Edition, 2005 Blackwell Publishing Inc.

Library of Congress Cataloging-in-Publication Data

Swanson, Todd A.
    Pathophysiology. II, GI, neurology, rheumatology, endocrinology / Todd Swanson, Sandra Kim, Olga E. Flomin.—5th ed.
        p. ; cm.—(Underground clinical vignettes)
    Rev. ed. of: Pathophysiology / Tao Le . . . [et al.]. 4th ed. c2005.
    Includes index.
    ISBN-13: 978-0-7817-6466-7
    ISBN-10: 0-7817-6466-1
    1. Physiology, Pathological—Case studies.   2. Physicians—Licenses—Examinations—Study guides.   I. Kim, Sandra.   II. Flomin, Olga E.   III. Pathophysiology.   IV. Title.
V. Title: GI, neurology, rheumatology, endocrinology.   VI. Series.
    [DNLM: 1. Clinical Medicine—Case Reports.   2. Clinical Medicine—Problems and Exercises.   WB 18.2 S9725pa 2007]
    RB113.B459 2007
    616.07076—dc22

                                                                2007001468

07 08 09 10
1 2 3 4 5 6 7 8 9 10

dedication

For T.M.

preface

First published in 1999, the Underground Clinical Vignettes (UCV) series has provided thousands of students with a highly effective review tool as they prepare for medical exams, particularly the USMLE Step 1 and 2 exams. Designed as a quick study guide, each UCV book contains patient-centered clinical cases that highlight a range of medical diagnoses.

With this new edition of Underground Clinical Vignettes, we have incorporated feedback from medical students across the country to provide updated cases with expanded treatment and discussion sections. A new two-page format enables readers to formulate an initial diagnosis prior to reading the answer, while the added differential diagnosis section encourages critical thinking about comparable cases. The inclusion of relevant MRI images, x-rays, and photographs allows students to visualize the physical presentation of each case more readily. Breakout boxes, tables, and algorithms have been added, along with all new Board-format QAs, making this edition of UCV an ideal source of information for exam review, classroom discussion, or clinical rotations.

The clinical vignettes in this series are designed to give added emphasis to pathogenesis, epidemiology, management, and complications. Although each case tends to present all the signs, symptoms, and diagnostic findings for a particular illness, patients generally will not present with such a "complete" picture either clinically or on a medical examination. Cases are not meant to simulate a potential real patient or an exam vignette.

Access to the LWW online companion site, ThePoint, is offered as a premium with the purchase of the Underground Clinical Vignettes Step 1 bundle. Benefits include an online test link and additional new Board-format questions covering all UCV subject areas.

We hope you will find the Underground Clinical Vignettes series informative and useful. We welcome any feedback, suggestions, or corrections you have about this series. Please contact us at LWW.com/medstudent.

contributors

Series Editors

Todd A. Swanson, M.D., Ph.D.
Resident in Radiation Oncology
William Beaumont Hospital
Royal Oak, Michigan

Sandra I. Kim, M.D., Ph.D.
Resident in Internal Medicine
Beth Israel Deaconess Medical Center
Harvard Medical School
Boston, Massachusetts

Series Contributors

Olga E. Flomin, M.D.
Resident in Obstetrics and Gynecology
William Beaumont Hospital
Royal Oak, Michigan

Medina C. Kushen, M.D.
Resident in Neurosurgery
University of Chicago Hospitals
Chicago, Illinois

Marc J. Glucksman, Ph.D.
Professor of Biochemistry and Molecular Biology
Director, Midwest Proteome Center and
Co-Director, Rosalind Franklin Structural Biology Laboratories
Rosalind Franklin University of Medicine and Science
The Chicago Medical School
North Chicago, Illinois

acknowledgments

Thanks to Dr. Alvaro Martinez, Dr. Larry Kestin and the entire radiation oncology program at William Beaumont Hospital for allowing the flexibility to work on this project during an already vigorous residency training program.

—Todd A. Swanson

Thanks to Todd for his work on this series.

—Sandra I. Kim

abbreviations

ABGs	arterial blood gases	BUN	blood urea nitrogen
ABPA	allergic bronchopulmonary aspergillosis	CABG	coronary artery bypass grafting
		CAD	coronary artery disease
ACA	anticardiolipin antibody	CaEDTA	calcium edetate
ACE	angiotensin-converting enzyme	CALLA	common acute lymphoblastic leukemia antigen
ACL	anterior cruciate ligament		
ACTH	adrenocorticotropic hormone	cAMP	cyclic adenosine monophosphate
AD	adjustment disorder		
ADA	adenosine deaminase	C-ANCA	cytoplasmic antineutrophil cytoplasmic antibody
ADD	attention-deficit disorder		
ADH	antidiuretic hormone	CBC	complete blood count
ADHD	attention-deficit–hyperactivity disorder	CBD	common bile duct
		CCU	cardiac care unit
ADP	adenosine diphosphate	CD	cluster of differentiation
AFO	ankle-foot orthosis	2-CdA	2-chlorodeoxyadenosine
AFP	α-fetoprotein	CEA	carcinoembryonic antigen
AIDS	acquired immunodeficiency syndrome	CFTR	cystic fibrosis transmembrane conductance regulator
ALL	acute lymphocytic leukemia	cGMP	cyclic guanosine monophosphate
ALS	amyotrophic lateral sclerosis		
ALT	alanine aminotransferase	CHF	congestive heart failure
AML	acute myelogenous leukemia	CK	creatine kinase
ANA	antinuclear antibody	CK-MB	creatine kinase, MB fraction
Angio	angiography	CLL	chronic lymphocytic leukemia
AP	anteroposterior	CML	chronic myelogenous leukemia
APKD	adult polycystic kidney disease	CMV	cytomegalovirus
aPTT	activated partial thromboplastin time	CN	cranial nerve
		CNS	central nervous system
ARDS	adult respiratory distress syndrome	COPD	chronic obstructive pulmonary disease
5-ASA	5-aminosalicylic acid	COX	cyclooxygenase
ASCA	antibodies to *Saccharomyces cerevisiae*	CP	cerebellopontine
		CPAP	continuous positive airway pressure
ASO	antistreptolysin O		
AST	aspartate aminotransferase	CPK	creatine phosphokinase
ATLL	adult T-cell leukemia/lymphoma	CPPD	calcium pyrophosphate dihydrate
ATPase	adenosine triphosphatase		
AV	arteriovenous, atrioventricular	CPR	cardiopulmonary resuscitation
AZT	azidothymidine (zidovudine)	CREST	calcinosis, Raynaud phenomenon, esophageal involvement, sclerodactyly, telangiectasia (syndrome)
BAL	British antilewisite (dimercaprol)		
BCG	bacillus Calmette-Guérin		
BE	barium enema		
BP	blood pressure	CRP	C-reactive protein
BPH	benign prostatic hypertrophy	CSF	cerebrospinal fluid

CSOM	chronic suppurative otitis media	EMG	electromyography
CT	cardiac transplant, computed tomography	ENT	ears, nose, and throat
		EPVE	early prosthetic valve endocarditis
CVA	cerebrovascular accident		
CXR	chest x-ray	ER	emergency room
d4T	didehydrodeoxythymidine (stavudine)	ERCP	endoscopic retrograde cholangiopancreatography
DCS	decompression sickness	ERT	estrogen replacement therapy
DDH	developmental dysplasia of the hip	ESR	erythrocyte sedimentation rate
		ETEC	enterotoxigenic *E. coli*
ddI	dideoxyinosine (didanosine)	EtOH	ethanol
DES	diethylstilbestrol	FAP	familial adenomatous polyposis
DEXA	dual-energy x-ray absorptiometry	FEV_1	forced expiratory volume in 1 second
DHEAS	dehydroepiandrosterone sulfate		
DIC	disseminated intravascular coagulation	FH	familial hypercholesterolemia
		FNA	fine-needle aspiration
DIF	direct immunofluorescence	FSH	follicle-stimulating hormone
DIP	distal interphalangeal (joint)	FTA-ABS	fluorescent treponemal antibody absorption test
DKA	diabetic ketoacidosis		
DL_{CO}	diffusing capacity of carbon monoxide	FVC	forced vital capacity
		G6PD	glucose-6-phosphate dehydrogenase
DMSA	2,3-dimercaptosuccinic acid		
DNA	deoxyribonucleic acid	GABA	gamma-aminobutyric acid
DNase	deoxyribonuclease	GERD	gastroesophageal reflux disease
2,3-DPG	2,3-diphosphoglycerate	GFR	glomerular filtration rate
dsDNA	double-stranded DNA	GGT	gamma-glutamyltransferase
DSM	Diagnostic and Statistical Manual	GH	growth hormone
		GI	gastrointestinal
dsRNA	double-stranded RNA	GnRH	gonadotropin-releasing hormone
DTP	diphtheria, tetanus, pertussis (vaccine)		
		GU	genitourinary
DTPA	diethylenetriamine-penta-acetic acid	GVHD	graft-versus-host disease
		HAART	highly active antiretroviral therapy
DTs	delirium tremens		
DVT	deep venous thrombosis	HAV	hepatitis A virus
EBV	Epstein–Barr virus	Hb	hemoglobin
ECG	electrocardiography	HbA-1C	hemoglobin A-1C
Echo	echocardiography	HBsAg	hepatitis B surface antigen
ECM	erythema chronicum migrans	HBV	hepatitis B virus
ECT	electroconvulsive therapy	hCG	human chorionic gonadotropin
EEG	electroencephalography	HCO_3	bicarbonate
EF	ejection fraction, elongation factor	Hct	hematocrit
		HCV	hepatitis C virus
EGD	esophagogastroduodenoscopy	HDL	high-density lipoprotein
EHEC	enterohemorrhagic *Escherichia coli*	HDL-C	high-density lipoprotein-cholesterol
EIA	enzyme immunoassay	HEENT	head, eyes, ears, nose, and throat (exam)
ELISA	enzyme-linked immunosorbent assay		
		HELLP	hemolysis, elevated LFTs, low platelets (syndrome)
EM	electron microscopy		

HFMD	hand, foot, and mouth disease	LDH	lactate dehydrogenase
HGPRT	hypoxanthine-guanine phospho-	LDL	low-density lipoprotein
	ribosyltransferase	LE	lupus erythematosus (cell)
5-HIAA	5-hydroxyindoleacetic acid	LES	lower esophageal sphincter
HIDA	hepato-iminodiacetic acid (scan)	LFTs	liver function tests
HIV	human immunodeficiency virus	LH	luteinizing hormone
HLA	human leukocyte antigen	LMN	lower motor neuron
HMG-CoA	hydroxymethylglutaryl-	LP	lumbar puncture
	coenzyme A	LPVE	late prosthetic valve
HMP	hexose monophosphate		endocarditis
HPI	history of present illness	L/S	lecithin/sphingomyelin (ratio)
HPV	human papillomavirus	LSD	lysergic acid diethylamide
HR	heart rate	LT	labile toxin
HRIG	human rabies immune globulin	LV	left ventricular
HRS	hepatorenal syndrome	LVH	left ventricular hypertrophy
HRT	hormone replacement therapy	Lytes	electrolytes
HSG	hysterosalpingography	Mammo	mammography
HSV	herpes simplex virus	MAO	monoamine oxidase (inhibitor)
HTLV	human T-cell leukemia virus	MCP	metacarpophalangeal (joint)
HUS	hemolytic-uremic syndrome	MCTD	mixed connective tissue
HVA	homovanillic acid		disorder
ICP	intracranial pressure	MCV	mean corpuscular volume
ICU	intensive care unit	MEN	multiple endocrine neoplasia
ID/CC	identification and chief	MI	myocardial infarction
	complaint	MIBG	meta-iodobenzylguanidine
IDDM	insulin-dependent diabetes		(radioisotope)
	mellitus	MMR	measles, mumps, rubella
IFA	immunofluorescent antibody		(vaccine)
Ig	immunoglobulin	MPGN	membranoproliferative
IGF	insulin-like growth factor		glomerulonephritis
IHSS	idiopathic hypertrophic	MPS	mucopolysaccharide
	subaortic stenosis	MPTP	1-methyl-4-phenyl-
IM	intramuscular		tetrahydropyridine
IMA	inferior mesenteric artery	MR	magnetic resonance (imaging)
INH	isoniazid	mRNA	messenger ribonucleic acid
INR	International Normalized Ratio	MRSA	methicillin-resistant *S. aureus*
IP_3	inositol 1,4,5-triphosphate	MTP	metatarsophalangeal (joint)
IPF	idiopathic pulmonary fibrosis	NAD	nicotinamide adenine
ITP	idiopathic thrombocytopenic		dinucleotide
	purpura	NADP	nicotinamide adenine
IUD	intrauterine device		dinucleotide phosphate
IV	intravenous	NADPH	reduced nicotinamide adenine
IVC	inferior vena cava		dinucleotide phosphate
IVIG	intravenous immunoglobulin	NF	neurofibromatosis
IVP	intravenous pyelography	NIDDM	non-insulin-dependent diabetes
JRA	juvenile rheumatoid arthritis		mellitus
JVP	jugular venous pressure	NNRTI	non-nucleoside reverse
KOH	potassium hydroxide		transcriptase inhibitor
KUB	kidney, ureter, bladder	NO	nitric oxide
LCM	lymphocytic choriomeningitis	NPO	nil per os (nothing by mouth)

NSAID	nonsteroidal anti-inflammatory drug	PO_2	partial pressure of oxygen
Nuc	nuclear medicine	PPD	purified protein derivative (of tuberculosis)
NYHA	New York Heart Association	PPH	primary postpartum hemorrhage
OB	obstetric		
OCD	obsessive–compulsive disorder	PRA	panel reactive antibody
OCPs	oral contraceptive pills	PROM	premature rupture of membranes
OR	operating room		
PA	posteroanterior	PSA	prostate-specific antigen
PABA	para-aminobenzoic acid	PSS	progressive systemic sclerosis
PAN	polyarteritis nodosa		
P-ANCA	perinuclear antineutrophil cytoplasmic antibody	PT	prothrombin time
		PTH	parathyroid hormone
PaO_2	partial pressure of oxygen in arterial blood	PTSD	posttraumatic stress disorder
		PTT	partial thromboplastin time
PAS	periodic acid Schiff	PUVA	psoralen ultraviolet A
PAT	paroxysmal atrial tachycardia	PVC	premature ventricular contraction
PBS	peripheral blood smear		
PCO_2	partial pressure of carbon dioxide	RA	rheumatoid arthritis
		RAIU	radioactive iodine uptake
PCOM	posterior communicating (artery)	RAST	radioallergosorbent test
		RBC	red blood cell
PCOS	polycystic ovarian syndrome	REM	rapid eye movement
PCP	phencyclidine	RES	reticuloendothelial system
PCR	polymerase chain reaction	RFFIT	rapid fluorescent focus inhibition test
PCT	porphyria cutanea tarda		
PCTA	percutaneous coronary transluminal angioplasty	RFTs	renal function tests
		RHD	rheumatic heart disease
PCV	polycythemia vera	RNA	ribonucleic acid
PDA	patent ductus arteriosus	RNP	ribonucleoprotein
PDGF	platelet-derived growth factor	RPR	rapid plasma reagin
PE	physical exam	RR	respiratory rate
PEFR	peak expiratory flow rate	RSV	respiratory syncytial virus
PEG	polyethylene glycol	RUQ	right upper quadrant
PEPCK	phosphoenolpyruvate carboxykinase	RV	residual volume
		SaO_2	oxygen saturation in arterial blood
PET	positron emission tomography		
PFTs	pulmonary function tests	SBFT	small bowel follow-through
PID	pelvic inflammatory disease	SCC	squamous cell carcinoma
PIP	proximal interphalangeal (joint)	SCID	severe combined immunodeficiency
PKU	phenylketonuria		
PMDD	premenstrual dysphoric disorder	SERM	selective estrogen receptor modulator
PML	progressive multifocal leukoencephalopathy	SGOT	serum glutamic-oxaloacetic transaminase
PMN	polymorphonuclear (leukocyte)	SIADH	syndrome of inappropriate antidiuretic hormone
PNET	primitive neuroectodermal tumor		
		SIDS	sudden infant death syndrome
PNH	paroxysmal nocturnal hemoglobinuria	SLE	systemic lupus erythematosus
		SMA	superior mesenteric artery

SSPE	subacute sclerosing panencephalitis
SSRI	selective serotonin-reuptake inhibitor
ST	stable toxin
STD	sexually transmitted disease
T2W	T2-weighted (MRI)
T_3	triiodothyronine
T_4	thyroxine
TAH-BSO	total abdominal hysterectomy–bilateral salpingo-oophorectomy
TB	tuberculosis
TCA	tricyclic antidepressant
TCC	transitional cell carcinoma
TDT	terminal deoxytransferase
TFTs	thyroid function tests
TGF	transforming growth factor
THC	tetrahydrocannabinol
TIA	transient ischemic attack
TLC	total lung capacity
TMP-SMX	trimethoprim-sulfamethoxazole
tPA	tissue plasminogen activator
TP-HA	*Treponema pallidum* hemagglutination assay
TPP	thiamine pyrophosphate
TRAP	tartrate-resistant acid phosphatase
tRNA	transfer ribonucleic acid
TSH	thyroid-stimulating hormone
TSS	toxic shock syndrome
TTP	thrombotic thrombocytopenic purpura
TURP	transurethral resection of the prostate
TXA	thromboxane A
UA	urinalysis
UDCA	ursodeoxycholic acid
UGI	upper GI
UPPP	uvulopalatopharyngoplasty
URI	upper respiratory infection
US	ultrasound
UTI	urinary tract infection
UV	ultraviolet
VDRL	Venereal Disease Research Laboratory
VIN	vulvar intraepithelial neoplasia
VIP	vasoactive intestinal polypeptide
VLDL	very low density lipoprotein
VMA	vanillylmandelic acid
V/Q	ventilation/perfusion (ratio)
VRE	vancomycin-resistant enterococcus
VS	vital signs
VSD	ventricular septal defect
vWF	von Willebrand factor
VZV	varicella-zoster virus
WAGR	Wilms tumor, aniridia, genitourinary abnormalities, mental retardation (syndrome)
WBC	white blood cell
WHI	Women's Health Initiative
WPW	Wolff–Parkinson–White syndrome
XR	x-ray
ZN	Ziehl–Neelsen (stain)

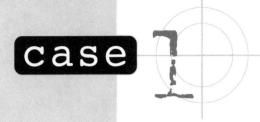

ID/CC	A 33-year-old woman complains of **increasing substernal pain and difficulty swallowing** liquids and solids (DYSPHAGIA) over the past several months.
HPI	She has lost 20 pounds in the past 3 months and has occasionally experienced acute substernal pain and **regurgitation of food** into her mouth when lying down.
PE	Unremarkable.
Labs	Esophageal manometry reveals aperistaltic esophagus; **increased lower esophageal sphincter pressure.**
Imaging	UGI: **"beak sign"** lower esophageal segment; **dilatation;** uncoordinated peristalsis. EGD: gaping cavity filled with dirty fluid. CXR: air-fluid level in enlarged esophagus.

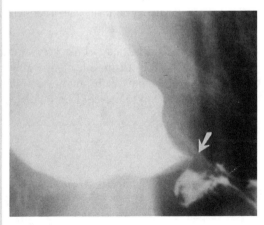

Figure 1-1. Bird beak sign

Gross Pathology	Massive dilatation of esophagus (due to defect in esophageal peristalsis and/or **impaired relaxation of lower esophageal sphincter** during swallowing).
Micro Pathology	Loss of number of ganglion cells in myenteric plexus (similar to Hirschsprung disease of the colon).

1

case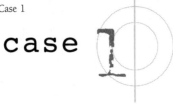

Achalasia

Differential

Esophageal carcinoma

Scleroderma

Chagas disease

Esophageal candidiasis

Diabetic gastroparesis

Gastric carcinoma

Discussion

Primary **idiopathic** achalasia is a motility disorder of the esophagus due to **loss of ganglion cells in myenteric plexus.** Complications include esophageal **squamous cell carcinoma,** candidal esophagitis, diverticula, and aspiration pneumonia. Secondary achalasia may be caused by **Chagas disease,** lymphoma, gastric carcinoma, or sarcoidosis. Achalasia may be part of autoimmune disorders, like scleroderma; however, such patients normally have a constellation of symptoms and are ANA positive.

Treatment

Calcium channel blockers; nitrates; endoscopic botulinum toxin injection; balloon dilatation; Heller myotomy with proton pump inhibitors or fundoplication to prevent later reflux.

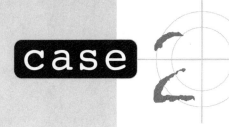

case

ID/CC A **34-year-old woman** presents to the ER with complaints of **colicky abdominal pain, spiking fever, and vomiting.**

HPI She was diagnosed with **gallstones** on an abdominal ultrasound several weeks ago and is awaiting elective surgery.

PE VS: fever (39.4°C); tachycardia (HR 120); tachypnea (RR 24); mild hypotension (BP 94/60). PE: **toxic-**looking patient; **scleral icterus** noted; **marked RUQ tenderness** with mild hepatomegaly on abdominal exam.

Labs CBC: **leukocytosis. Markedly elevated direct bilirubin and alkaline phosphatase** with moderately elevated AST and ALT; normal albumin, PT, and PTT; **blood cultures** positive for *Escherichia coli.*

Imaging **US, abdomen: dilated common bile duct (CBD) with obstructing stone.** CT, abdomen: gallstones and stone in CBD with dilated intrahepatic bile ducts.

case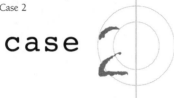

Ascending Cholangitis

Differential	Primary sclerosing cholangitis
	Cholecystitis
	Hepatitis
	Pancreatitis
	Mesenteric ischemia
Discussion	Prolonged choledocholithiasis leads to suppurative cholangitis, which has a very high mortality rate.

Breakout Point

Cholangitis Presents with Reynold Pentad

1. Right upper quadrant pain
2. Fever
3. Jaundice
4. Central nervous system symptoms
5. Septic shock

Treatment — **NPO** with nasogastric suction; **IV antibiotics**; emergent endoscopic (interventional ERCP) or surgical **biliary tree decompression** followed by laparoscopic or open **cholecystectomy**.

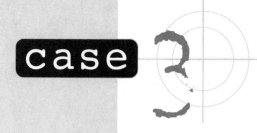

ID/CC A 50-year-old man presents with a long-standing history of **retrosternal burning, belching, and water brash,** especially after meals.

HPI He is a **chronic smoker and alcoholic** and is under treatment for **gastroesophageal reflux dyspepsia.**

PE Physical exam normal.

Labs UGI endoscopy reveals linear streaks of red, velvety mucosa at gastroesophageal junction.

Imaging Barium swallow: fine reticular pattern distal to an esophageal stricture; gastroesophageal reflux.

Gross Pathology **Red, velvety mucosa in form of circumferential band and linear streaks around gastroesophageal junction.**

Micro Pathology Mixture of **metaplastic gastric and intestinal-type columnar epithelial cells** (mucin-secreting and absorptive, respectively).

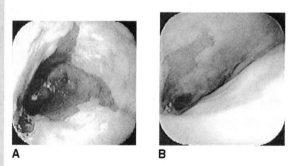

A   **B**

Figure 3-1. A microscopic section of the metaplastic epithelium shows a villiform surface with numerous goblet cells.

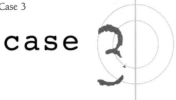

case

Barrett Esophagus

Differential

Esophagitis

Gastrointestinal reflux disease

Esophageal cancer

Discussion

Barrett esophagus is marked by **metaplasia of the distal esophageal squamous epithelium to a columnar epithelium in response to prolonged injury;** long-standing esophageal reflux leads to inflammation and ulceration of squamous mucosa. Healing occurs through re-epithelialization by pluripotent cells, which in the setting of low pH differentiates into the more resistant gastric (both cardiac and fundic) type or the specialized columnar (intestinal) type. Only the columnar type is clinically important. The most serious complication is the development of **adenocarcinoma;** hence, patients with Barrett esophagus should undergo endoscopic surveillance every 2 to 3 years. Additional complications of Barrett esophagus may include stricture formation and ulcerations.

Treatment

Proton pump inhibitors, H_2 antagonists, and antacids; cessation of smoking and alcohol; careful endoscopic follow-up to detect esophageal cancer.

case

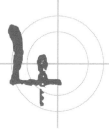

ID/CC	A 40-year-old woman is seen with complaints of sudden-onset, progressively increasing **abdominal distention and pain** and **vomiting**.
HPI	The patient also complains of **visible abdominal and back veins** that appear while she is **standing** and **look like ropes**. In addition, she has observed **increasing swelling of her feet**. She has been taking **oral contraceptives** for a few years.
PE	Icterus; **pitting pedal edema**; markedly distended abdomen; dilated, tortuous veins over abdomen and back; **hepatojugular reflux absent**; fluid thrill but shifting dullness present (ascites); mildly tender **hepatomegaly** and **splenomegaly**.
Labs	CBC: leukocytosis. LFTs elevated; ascitic fluid **transudative**.
Imaging	US, abdomen: hepatosplenomegaly and ascites. US, Doppler: increased portal vein flow; **hepatic veins obstructed where they empty into the inferior vena cava**. IVC portovenography: confirms obstruction.
Gross Pathology	Thrombosis of hepatic vein where it drains into the inferior vena cava. Liver is swollen, reddish purple, and has a tense capsule.

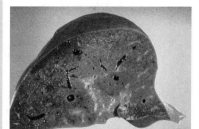

Figure 4-1. The cut surface of the liver shows thrombosis of the hepatic veins and diffuse congestion of the parenchyma.

Micro Pathology	Affected areas show severe centrilobular congestion and necrosis along with sinusoidal dilatation.

7

case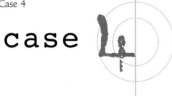

Budd–Chiari Syndrome

Differential

Constrictive pericarditis
Right-sided heart failure
Metastatic liver cancer
Alcoholic liver disease

Treatment

Balloon angioplasty with stent; surgical removal or bypass of the obstruction; life-long anticoagulation; **cessation of oral contraceptives;** diuretics along with sodium and fluid restriction.

Discussion

Budd–Chiari syndrome occurs with conditions that predispose to thrombosis, e.g., polycythemia vera, pregnancy, postpartum states, use of oral contraceptives, paroxysmal nocturnal hemoglobinuria (PNH), and intra-abdominal cancers; membranous webs in the inferior vena cava. Untreated Budd–Chiari syndrome may progress to liver failure.

case 5

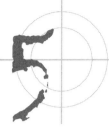

ID/CC	A 45-year-old man who has been diagnosed with **AIDS** presents with **pain on swallowing** (ODYNOPHAGIA) and mild **difficulty swallowing** (DYSPHAGIA).
HPI	These symptoms are markedly aggravated by the ingestion of acidic fluids.
PE	**Oral thrush.**
Labs	Culture of esophageal washings reveals *Candida albicans*.
Imaging	Esophagoscopy: small, raised **white or yellow plaques.**
Gross Pathology	Scattered yellowish white plaques with occasional mucosal ulcers.
Micro Pathology	Cytologic examination of brushings reveals presence of yeast cells.

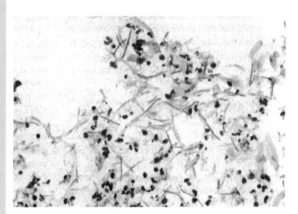

Figure 5-1. Close-up view of the plaque material demonstrates mycelia and spores.

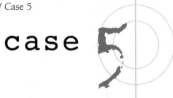

case

Candida Esophagitis

Differential
Herpes esophagitis
CMV esophagitis
HIV esophagitis
Gastrointestinal reflux
Chemical burns

Discussion
The current surge in candidal esophageal infections is due to AIDS and to post-organ-transplant immuno-suppression therapy. However, even individuals with mild immunosuppression such as those with diabetes can have candida esophagitis.

Treatment
Usually in minimally immunocompromised patients nystatin or clotrimazole are used. However, in patients with AIDS ketoconazole and fluconazole are used. In the event of refractory cases, amphotericin can be used.

case 6

ID/CC A 12-year-old white girl, the daughter of **Norwegian** immigrants, complains of **diarrhea and flatulence.**

HPI Her parents say she has suffered from weight loss despite that she eats well. Her mother adds that her stool is **foul-smelling** and **greasy** (STEATORRHEA) with no blood or mucus.

PE Pale and thin; xerosis (DRYNESS) and hyperkeratosis of skin (due to vitamin A malabsorption); pruritic, erythematous vesicular rash on knees, elbows, and neck; cheilosis (SCALING); ecchymoses.

Labs CBC: macrocytic, hypochromic anemia. Lytes: decreased potassium and calcium. **Elevated serum antigliadin** and **anti-endomysial antibodies.** Decreased serum cholesterol and albumin; prolonged PT; **abnormal d-xylose test;** positive Sudan stain for fecal fat.

Imaging UGI/SBFT: loss of mucosal folds and **dilated jejunum.**

Micro Pathology Hallmark **flattening and atrophy of mucosal villi** with basophilia and loss of nuclear polarity; lymphocytic and plasma cell infiltration of lamina propria.

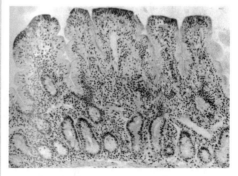

Figure 6-1. Note the blunted, shortened villus, the intra-epithelial lymphocytes in the surface epithelium, and the prominent infiltrate of lymphocytes and plasma cells in the lamina propria.

11

case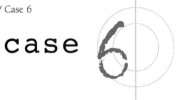

Celiac Disease

Differential

Bacterial overgrowth
Crohn disease
Eosinophilic gastroenteritis
Infectious gastroenteritis
Irritable bowel syndrome
Giardiasis

Discussion

Celiac disease is a disease of the small intestine that is due to **gluten** (gliadin) **hypersensitivity.** It is associated with HLA-DR3 and HLA-DQw2 and is characterized by varying degrees of **nutrient malabsorption:** iron, folate, fat-soluble vitamins (A, D, E, K). It is also known as **nontropical sprue, celiac sprue,** or gluten-sensitive enteropathy. Patients often have an associated skin rash known as dermatitis hepetiformis. Ecchymoses can result from vitamin K malabsorption/deficiency.

Treatment

Gluten-free diet is both diagnostic and therapeutic, glucocorticoids for refractory cases.

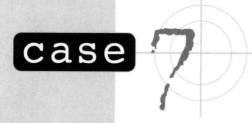

case 7

ID/CC   A **66-year-old Scandinavian** man comes to the doctor's office for an insurance physical complaining of increasing **fatigue, occasional indigestion, and diarrhea.**

HPI   He has been taking antacids for his dyspepsia.

PE   **Marked pallor; mild splenomegaly.**

Labs   CBC/PBS: **macrocytic anemia,** macro-ovalocytes, and hypersegmented neutrophils. Low vitamin B_{12} levels; elevated homocystine and methylmalonic acid; **Schilling test confirms vitamin B_{12} malabsorption** corrected with administration of intrinsic factor; **antiparietal cell antibodies present; reduced gastric acid formation** (ACHLORHYDRIA).

Imaging   Endoscopy: thinning of mucosa and flattening of rugal fold seen more in fundus and body of stomach with **sparing of antrum.**

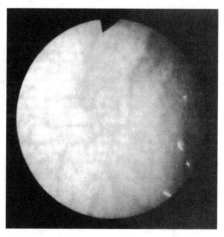

Figure 7-1. Thinning of mucosa and flattening of rugal fold seen.

Micro Pathology   Lymphocytes and plasma cell infiltrates in lamina propria; decreased number of glands.

13

case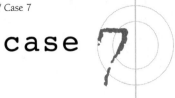

Chronic Atrophic Gastritis

Differential

Gastroesophageal reflux disease
Crohn disease
Peptic ulcer disease
B-cell lymphoma

Discussion

Pernicious anemia is characterized by chronic atrophic gastritis with achlorhydria and antibodies to parietal cells and intrinsic factor. The condition is more common among older patients (mean age of 60); these patients are predisposed to other autoimmune disorders, such as vitiligo, hypoparathyroidism, adrenal insufficiency, and thyroid disease.

Treatment

Parenteral administration of vitamin B_{12}; regular follow-up (chronic atrophic gastritis **predisposes to gastric carcinoma**).

case 8

ID/CC A 45-year-old **alcoholic** man presents with **recurrent epigastric pain** that sometimes radiates to his back.

HPI He also complains of **bulky, greasy, foul-smelling stool** (STEATORRHEA). He has **lost 10 pounds** over the past 3 months.

PE **Epigastric pain** on deep palpation.

Labs Quantitative estimation of fat in stool reveals **steatorrhea; elevated serum amylase and lipase levels.**

Imaging XR, abdomen: **pancreatic calcification.** CT/US: **pancreatic atrophy and calcification.** ERCP: small stricture of pancreatic duct in head; distal pancreatic duct shows sacculation with intervening **short strictures** ("CHAIN OF LAKES").

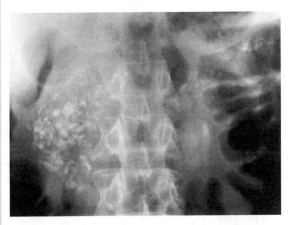

Figure 8-1. Multiple, scattered, small concretions in the pancreas.

Gross Pathology **Scarred-down, fibrotic pancreas** with whitish areas of fatty necrosis and areas of **cystic cavitation.**

Micro Pathology Pancreatic biopsy reveals presence of dilated ducts, fibrotic stroma, and atrophy of exocrine glands and islets (due to enzymatic fat necrosis).

15

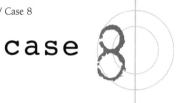

case 8

Chronic Pancreatitis

Differential

Cholangitis
Crohn disease
Chronic gastritis
Pancreatic cancer
Myocardial infarction

Discussion

Chronic pancreatitis is a persistent inflammatory disease of the pancreas that is irreversible and causes pain and permanent impairment of endocrine and exocrine function. **Alcohol abuse** is the most common cause in **adults, cystic fibrosis in children.**

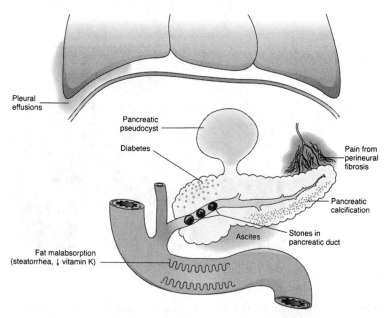

Figure 8-2. Complications of chronic pancreatitis.

Treatment

Pancreatic **enzyme replacement; low-fat diet;** surgery for relief of intractable pain.

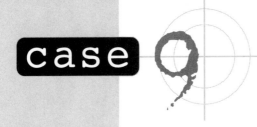

case 9

ID/CC A 61-year-old white man in apparent good health has a routine annual physical exam that reveals a small rectal mass.

HPI He has no major complaints except for intermittent, mild diarrhea.

PE **Mobile, nonpainful rectal mass** on digital rectal exam with no evidence of bleeding; examination otherwise unremarkable.

Labs CBC: **anemia** (Hb 9.2/Hct 26.9). **Hemoccult-positive stool.**

Imaging Sigmoidoscopy/BE: multiple **pedunculated masses** in sigmoid and transverse colon.

Gross Pathology Discrete mass lesions from colonic epithelium protruding into intestinal lumen; vast majority measure <2 cm, although may reach up to 5 cm; may have stalk (PEDUNCULATED) or have a broad base (SESSILE); may be **tubular, villous,** or **tubulovillous.**

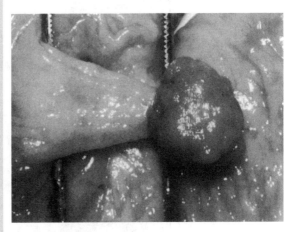

Figure 9-1. Pedunculated mass in the colon.

Micro Pathology Frequent mitosis, cellular atypia, and loss of normal polarity in intestinal epithelium of glands.

17

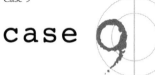

case 9

Colonic Polyps

Differential

Colon cancer
Intestinal leiomyosarcoma
Rectal cancer
Lipomas
Peutz–Jeghers syndrome

Discussion

The **oncogene** associated with adenomatous polyposis coli is the **tumor suppressor gene** located on **chromosome 5**. The most common variety is adenomatous; the **risk of malignant transformation increases with size, villous** morphology, and the **familial** form of the disease (which has a 100% probability of becoming malignant).

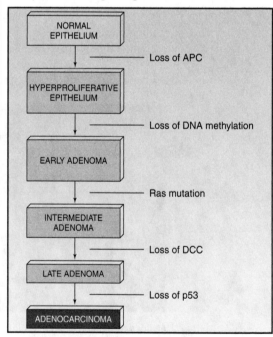

Figure 9-2. Adenoma–carcinoma sequence.

Treatment

Colonoscopic biopsy and removal; repeat colonoscopy or barium enema for periodic surveillance.

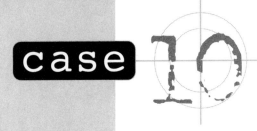

ID/CC A 21-year-old woman complains of **intermittent abdominal pain, mild, nonbloody diarrhea,** and anorexia of 2 year duration.

HPI She says that the pain is almost always confined to the **right lower abdomen** and is cramping in nature.

PE Pallor; weight loss; **abdominal mass in right iliac fossa** (thickened bowel loop); **perianal fistulas.**

Labs CBC: megaloblastic anemia. **Guaiac positive;** stool negative for parasites.

Imaging BE: granulomatous colitis and **regional enteritis** involving multiple areas, most commonly ileum and ascending colon.

Gross Pathology **Terminal ileum** (lesions most commonly seen in ileocecal) shows lesions that have a "cobblestone" appearance; **discontinuous areas of inflammation, edema, and fibrosis** ("SKIP LESIONS").

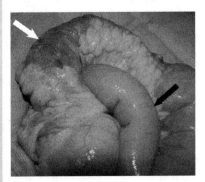

Figure 10-1. Normal ileum (light arrow); affected terminal ileum (dark arrow).

Micro Pathology **Chronic inflammatory involvement of submucosal layers of bowel wall** (TRANSMURAL INFLAMMATION), manifested mainly by lymphocytic infiltration with associated lymphoid hyperplasia and formation of noncaseating granulomas.

19

case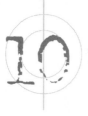

Crohn Disease

Differential

Appendicitis
Clostridium difficile colitis
Ulcerative colitis
Diverticulitis
Viral gastroenteritis
Celiac sprue

Discussion

Complications of Crohn disease include adhesions, ulcers, strictures, fissures, and fistulas. Extra-intestinal manifestations may include arthritis, ankylosing spondylitis, sclerosing cholangitis, and uveitis. Patients with Crohn disease also have a five- to six-fold increased risk of developing colon cancer; however, this risk is much lower than that associated with ulcerative colitis.

Treatment

Antidiarrheal drugs and systemic glucocorticoids; 5-aminosalicylic acid agents (e.g., sulfasalazine); antimetabolites such as azathioprine or mercaptopurine in patients with fistulous disease; antitumor necrosis factor antibody for refractory disease; **surgery** if patients develop severe malabsorption, symptomatic fistulas, or subacute intestinal obstruction.

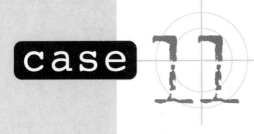

case 11

GASTROINTESTINAL

ID/CC A 54-year-old white woman complains of **colicky pain in the left lower abdomen** and **fever.**

HPI She has had **frequent attacks of moderate pain** in the same area for several months and one episode of **bloody stools** without excessive mucus.

PE VS: low-grade fever. PE: pallor; tenderness; rebound and guarding of left lower quadrant but normal stools; **sigmoid colon palpable, thickened, and tender.**

Labs CBC: **normocytic, normochromic anemia; neutrophilic leukocytosis** with associated left shift (BANDEMIA). Stool culture reveals no pathogens.

Imaging Pericolonic inflammatory stranding: **"saw-toothed" appearance.**

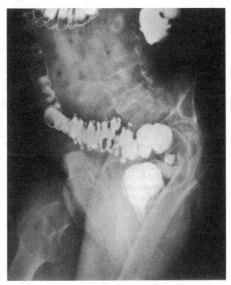

Figure 11-1. Saw toothing of sigmoid colon.

Gross Pathology Resected segment reveals external **outpouchings** up to 1 cm in diameter along colon between tenia coli **from lumen; small mucosal openings lead into pouches.**

21

case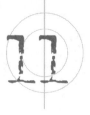

Diverticulitis

Differential

Appendicitis
Constipation
Inflammatory bowel disease
Mesenteric ischemia
Pyelonephritis
Nephrolithiasis

Discussion

Diverticulitis is a condition of the colon in which the mucosa and submucosa herniate through the muscular layers of the colon to form outpouchings that may become obstructed with feces. The pathogenesis involves **increased intraluminal pressure** and **focal weakness** of the wall of the colon (near areas of nerve and vessel penetration alongside the taeniae coli). Outpouchings may become repeatedly inflamed, resulting in **abscess** formation, development of **fistulas** to adjoining organs, colonic obstruction, perforation, and sepsis. It is most commonly seen in the **sigmoid colon.**

Treatment

High-fiber diet; antibiotics for diverticulitis; surgical resection of severely involved segments.

case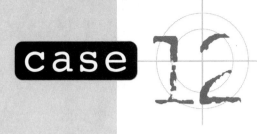

ID/CC	A **60-year-old** woman presents with **lower abdominal discomfort, chronic constipation**, and **passage of bright red blood per rectum.**
HPI	She is a heavy smoker, and her diet contains a significant amount of greasy food and **little natural fiber.**
PE	VS: normal. PE: pallor; mild left lower abdominal tenderness with **palpable descending colon; guaiac-positive** stool on rectal exam.
Labs	CBC: normocytic, normochromic anemia. **Frank blood in stool; no leukocytes or epithelial cells** seen.
Imaging	Sigmoidoscopy: **multiple small outpouchings** in walls of **descending** and **sigmoid colon** without inflammation.
Gross Pathology	Multiple subcentimeter flasklike outpouchings alongside taeniae coli in walls of descending and sigmoid colon.
Micro Pathology	Thin-walled herniations of atrophic mucosa and compressed submucosa; hypertrophied circular layer of muscularis propria with prominent taeniae coli.

case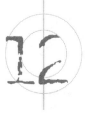

Diverticulosis

Differential

Fecal impaction
Colon cancer
Infectious colitis
Ischemic colitis
Meckel diverticula

Discussion

Diverticuli are outpouchings in the colonic walls in which the arteries penetrate the muscularis layer to reach the mucosal wall, creating an inherently weak area. Most commonly found in the descending and sigmoid colon, diverticulosis is a disease of **Western industrialized society,** with a **low-fiber/high-fat diet** a significant contributory factor. Complications include inflammation of the diverticuli (DIVERTICULITIS), significant lower GI bleeding, perforation, abscess formation, and colovesical fistula.

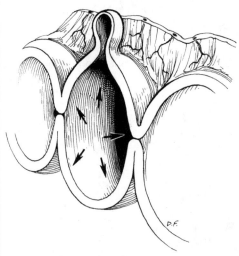

Figure 12-1. Formation of diverticula.

Treatment

High dietary fiber; supplement diet with soluble fiber and bulk-forming laxatives such as **psyllium;** surgery for management of recurrent heavy diverticular bleeding.

case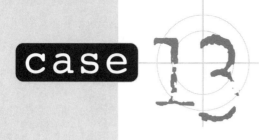

ID/CC A 35-year-old woman presents with **difficulty swallowing.**

HPI She also complains of **retrosternal chest pain and heartburn.** She is not currently taking any medications, is a nonsmoker, and drinks alcohol only occasionally.

PE VS: normal. PE: normal.

Labs CBC: normal. ESR, ANA, RA factor: normal. ECG: normal.

Imaging Esophagogram: multiple, simultaneous esophageal contractions (like a **giant corkscrew**). Esophageal manometry: lower part of esophagus demonstrates prolonged, **nonsequential, large-amplitude, repetitive contractions of simultaneous onset.**

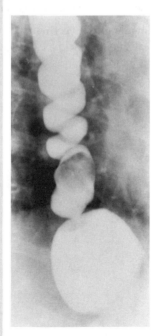

Figure 13-1. Corkscrew appearance of esophagus.

25

case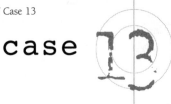

Esophageal Spasm

Differential

Achalasia
Angina pectoris
Esophageal diverticula
Esophageal stricture
Esophageal webs and rings
Esophagitis

Discussion

Esophageal spasm is characterized by **uncoordinated esophageal muscle contractions** that do not propel food into the stomach. Esophageal spasm is seen in association with **advanced age, emotional stress**, collagen vascular disease, reflux esophagitis, esophageal obstruction, and irradiation esophagitis. Pain due to esophageal spasm **mimics angina**, which should be included in the differential diagnosis.

Treatment

Sublingual nitroglycerin for acute attacks; anxiolytics and calcium channel blockers; H$_2$ blockers or proton pump inhibitors for associated GERD; myotomy for refractory disease.

case 14

ID/CC	A 47-year-old white **man** is brought by ambulance to the emergency room because of **massive, painless vomiting of bright red blood** (HEMATEMESIS) and shock.
HPI	He is a known homeless **alcoholic** who lives in the streets surrounding the hospital. His friend states that he has been drinking heavily for the past 2 months.
PE	VS: **tachycardia; hypotension.** PE: skin cold and clammy; **hard nodular hepatomegaly;** mild **splenomegaly;** spider nevi; caput medusae; clubbing; ascites, mild gynecomastia; bilaterally enlarged parotid glands.
Labs	CBC/PBS: normocytic, normochromic **anemia.** Low serum albumin; **elevated alkaline phosphatase; increased bilirubin, ALT, AST.**
Imaging	EGD: actively bleeding along the esophagus.
Gross Pathology	**Tortuous** and **dilated submucosal esophageal veins** secondary to shunting from **portal hypertension;** superficial ulceration, inflammation, and rupture.

case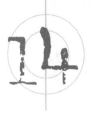

Esophageal Variceal Bleeding

Differential

Gastric ulcer

Mallory–Weiss tear

Esophagitis

Angiodysplasia

Aortoenteric fistula

Discussion

Esophageal varices are often silent until they rupture and are associated with a significant mortality rate. **Cirrhosis** is the most common cause, but other causes of portal hypertension may also be involved, including Budd–Chiari syndrome, tumor invasion of the portal vein, and metabolic diseases that alter liver sinusoids (e.g., amyloid).

Treatment

Restore blood volume, vasoconstrictors (e.g., vaso-pressin, octreotide), balloon tamponade of varices followed by endoscopic sclerotherapy; splenorenal or transjugular intrahepatic portosystemic shunt (TIPS) if sclerotherapy fails; propranolol for chronic treat-ment of portal hypertension.

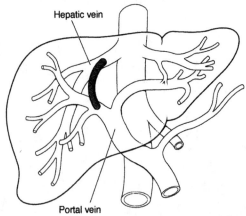

Figure 14-1. The TIPS is a metal expandable stent that is placed angiographically between branches of the hepatic and portal veins to create a nonsurgical shunt between the portal and systemic venous systems.

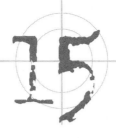

case 15

ID/CC A 35-year-old **obese** man who is a **chronic smoker** presents with **heartburn.**

HPI His heartburn **worsens** when bending and **lying down at night,** preventing him from sleeping; it is promptly **relieved with antacids.**

Labs Continuous esophageal pH monitoring correlates symptoms with posture, meals, and reflux.

Imaging UGI: small **hiatal hernia; spontaneous reflux** to mid-esophagus. EGD: erythema, friability, and erosions over esophageal mucosa.

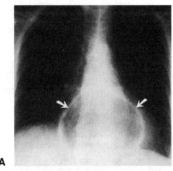

A

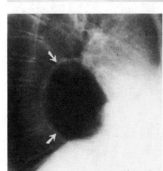

B

Figure 15-1. A large hiatal hernia is present.

Micro Pathology Evidence of inflammation on biopsy; no malignant change noted.

29

case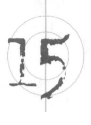

Gastroesophageal Reflux Disease

Differential

Barrett esophagus

Esophageal carcinoma

Gastric ulcer

Hiatal hernia

Gastroparesis

Discussion

The pathophysiology of gastroesophageal reflux disease (GERD) involves a sustained **decrease in LES tone** (caused by muscle weakness, scleroderma-like diseases, pregnancy, smoking, alcohol, or surgery), which allows reflux to occur. The extent of damage depends on the amount of refluxed material per episode, the frequency of episodes, the clearance rate by gravity and peristalsis, and the rate of neutralization of acids by salivary secretion. Chronic untreated GERD can lead to stricture formation or columnar metaplasia of distal esophagus epithelium (BARRETT ESOPHAGUS), which predisposes to esophageal **adenocarcinoma.**

Treatment

Cessation of smoking; elevation of head of bed; weight reduction; avoidance of fatty foods, coffee, chocolate, and alcohol; **H$_2$ receptor antagonists, proton pump inhibitors,** and **antacids** provide symptomatic relief; metoclopramide increases lower esophageal sphincter pressure and speeds gastric emptying, preventing reflux; surgery (e.g., Nissen fundoplication).

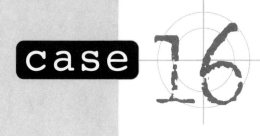

case 16

ID/CC A 50-year-old **Caucasian** man presents with progressively increasing **yellowing of the eyes** (JAUNDICE), a peculiar **skin rash**, and **palpitations**.

HPI On directed questioning, he admits to having **decreased libido.** Three years ago he was diagnosed with **diabetes** and is on oral hypoglycemics. He smokes and drinks alcohol only occasionally, has never received a blood transfusion, and has no prior history of jaundice.

PE Generalized **bronze discoloration** of skin; irregular pulse; icterus; loss of pubic and axillary hair; testicular atrophy; firm, nontender, nonpulsatile hepatomegaly.

Labs Increased blood glucose; elevated LFTs; decreased serum testosterone and gonadotropins; **increased serum iron; decreased total iron-binding capacity; transferrin saturation <50%; serum ferritin >300 μg/L (best screening method)**; genetic testing positive for two HFE mutations (C282Y, H63D). ECG: **atrial fibrillation.**

Imaging CT, abdomen: diffusely increased liver density. Echo: **cardiomyopathy.**

Gross Pathology Liver shows pigmentary cirrhosis.

Micro Pathology Cirrhosis with abundant hemosiderin deposition in liver cells, Kupffer cells, and bile ducts.

case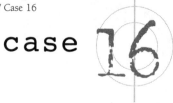

Hereditary Hemochromatosis

Differential

β-Thalassemia

Bantu siderosis

Transfusion hemosiderosis

Zellweger syndrome

Alcoholic liver disease

Porphyrias

Discussion

In idiopathic hemochromatosis, iron accumulates until the total body iron content reaches 50 g. The cause is a breakdown in the normal control of iron absorption from the GI tract due to HFE gene mutation; normally, the amount of iron accumulated inversely affects the GI mucosal absorption of both heme and nonheme iron. As iron overload progresses, iron that is ordinarily stored in the cells of the reticuloendothelial system is deposited in the liver, joints, gonads, pancreas, heart, and skin.

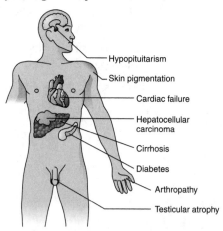

Hypopituitarism

Skin pigmentation

Cardiac failure

Hepatocellular carcinoma

Cirrhosis

Diabetes

Arthropathy

Testicular atrophy

Figure 16-1. Complications of hemochromatosis.

Treatment

Repeated phlebotomies; avoidance of alcohol; monitor for development of **hepatoma** (due to increased risk); liver transplantation for end-stage disease; **screen first-degree relatives.**

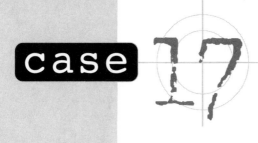

case 17

ID/CC A 50-year-old man with a history of **alcoholism** is unresponsive to stimuli when brought by a neighbor to the emergency room.

HPI His neighbor states that he had **vomited blood** (HEMATEMESIS) 3 months ago but had received no treatment. The neighbor also says that the patient got drunk three times a week for 4 years until approximately 1 year ago.

PE Muscle wasting; **icteric sclera; spider angiomata** (due to increased levels of estrogen); nodular, **hard hepatomegaly; caput medusae;** loss of hair on chest and genitalia; **ascites;** gynecomastia; testicular atrophy; parotid enlargement; **flapping tremor of hands** (ASTERIXIS); **palmar erythema;** slight pitting edema in lower extremities.

Labs CBC/PBS: slight thrombocytopenia; macrocytic anemia. Increased bilirubin; elevated serum transaminase and alkaline phosphatase; **low serum albumin** with increased globulins; **prolonged PT; high blood ammonia.**

Imaging UGI: **esophageal varices.** EGD: esophageal varices confirmed. CT/US, abdomen: enlarged and fatty liver; tortuous, dilated variceal vessels.

Gross Pathology Early: enlargement and fatty infiltration of liver; late: brownish discoloration, hardening, and atrophy of liver parenchyma.

Micro Pathology Necrosis of normal hepatocytes; diffuse replacement with fibrous connective tissue and lymphocyte infiltrate; **regenerating nodules of liver lacking normal organization;** eosinophilic Mallory bodies; bile congested ductules and proliferation of fibroblasts.

case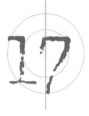

Hepatic Cirrhosis

Differential

Hepatocellular carcinoma
Portal vein thrombosis
Congestive heart failure
Hepatitis

Discussion

Hepatic cirrhosis is most commonly caused by alcohol; less commonly it is caused by biliary diseases, hepatitis B and C, Wilson disease, and hemochromatosis. End-stage liver disease leads to liver failure, nutritional deficiencies, GI bleeding, and toxic ammonemia. There is also an increased risk of hepatocellular carcinoma.

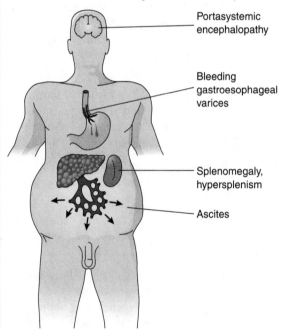

Figure 17-1. Complications of cirrhosis.

Treatment

Discontinue alcohol; supportive treatment of ascites, encephalopathy, variceal bleeding, and anemia; evaluation for liver transplantation in selected cases.

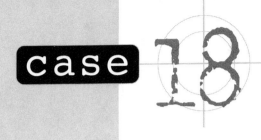

case 18

ID/CC A 56-year-old man with yellowing of the eyes and skin (due to **severe jaundice**) is brought to the ER in an **agitated state**.

HPI He has been passing black, tarry, foul-smelling stools (MELENA) and has exhibited a **reversal of sleep pattern** with **daytime sleepiness**. A few months ago he **vomited blood** (HEMATEMESIS) and was admitted to the hospital, at which time he was diagnosed with **alcoholic liver cirrhosis.**

PE VS: tachycardia; tachypnea; hypotension. PE: **lethargic and somnolent**; marked **icterus; feculent, fruity breath** (FETOR HEPATICUS); signs of chronic liver disease found; asterixis, dysarthria, and primitive reflexes (suck and snout) demonstrated; exaggerated deep tendon reflexes; **ascites; liver span reduced; splenomegaly.**

Labs **LFTs markedly elevated** (increased serum bilirubin, AST, and ALT; decreased serum albumin, reversed albumin-to-globulin ratio); alkaline phosphatase moderately elevated; prolonged PT; elevated serum ammonia. EEG: symmetric slowing; triphasic waves.

Imaging Endoscopy (during previous admission): **bleeding esophageal varices.**

case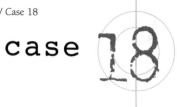

Hepatic Encephalopathy

Differential

Hepatocellular carcinoma

Portal vein thrombosis

Congestive heart failure

Hepatitis

Discussion

The postulated mechanisms for the development of hepatic encephalopathy include **elevated concentrations of blood ammonia, short-chain fatty acids, false neurotransmitters,** decreased branched-chain amino acids, and a circulating substance that has properties similar to that of benzodiazepine agonists that potentiate the action of **GABA.**

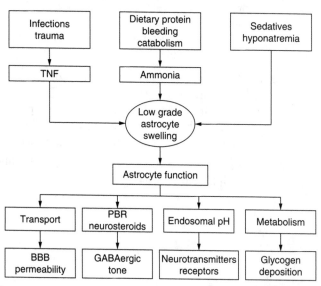

Figure 18-1. Proposed mechanism through which various precipitating factors can induce hepatic encephalopathy.

Treatment

Eliminate precipitating factors (such as GI bleeding, electrolyte imbalance, and infection); **low-protein diet; neomycin** and **lactulose** (induces diarrhea and clears the gut; alters bowel flora; and converts NH_3 to NH_4 which is less absorbable).

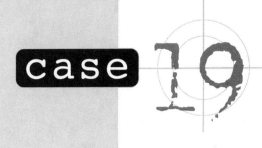

case 19

ID/CC	A 40-year-old **man** presents with complaints of increasing **yellowness** of his eyes and skin, **darkly colored urine**, and loss of appetite.
HPI	He has no history of blood transfusions, contact with other jaundiced persons, or exposure to an epidemic of hepatitis in the neighborhood; the patient is a known **alcoholic**.
PE	Fever; **icterus**; parotid enlargement; **Dupuytren contracture** in left index and little finger; **palmar erythema**; mildly **tender hepatomegaly**; no splenomegaly or ascites.
Labs	CBC: microcytic anemia; leukocytosis. Elevated serum bilirubin; **elevated AST and ALT** (AST > ALT, usually by a factor of two) (typically seen in alcoholic liver disease; in other parenchymal liver diseases, ALT is more elevated); increased alkaline phosphatase and γ-glutamyltransferase (GGT); serologic markers negative for hepatitis A, B, and C; PT prolonged.
Imaging	US, abdomen: hepatomegaly with coarsened echo texture suggestive of hepatitis and fatty infiltration.
Gross Pathology	Enlarged liver with yellow and greasy surface (shrunken size with micronodular surface is seen in cirrhotic stage).
Micro Pathology	**Hepatocellular necrosis, neutrophilic infiltration, and alcoholic hyaline bodies** (MALLORY BODIES); some hepatocytes distended with fat, displacing nucleus to side; perivenular and sinusoidal fibrosis also seen.

case

Hepatitis—Alcoholic

Differential

Hepatitis B

Hepatitis C

Chronic pancreatitis

Discussion

Liver diseases produced by excessive consumption of ethanol include fatty liver, alcoholic hepatitis, and cirrhosis; fatty change and, to an extent, alcoholic hepatitis may reverse fully with abstinence. Approximately 10% to 15% of chronic alcoholics develop cirrhosis. The severity of alcoholic hepatitis can range from mild illness to fulminant hepatic failure. The severity of liver disease can be quantified by Child–Pugh score.

■ **TABLE 19-1 CHILD–PUGH SCORE**

	Points		
Criterion	1	2	3
Serum bilirubin (mg/dL)	<2	2–3	>3
Serum albumin (g/dL)	>3.5	3–3.5	<3
Ascites	None	Easily controlled	Poorly controlled
Encephalopathy	None	Minimal	Advanced
Prothrombin time (INR)	<1.7	1.7–2.3	>2.3

Note: 5–6 points, Child–Pugh class A; 7–9 points, Child–Pugh class B; 10–15 points, Child–Pugh class C. INR, international normalized ratio.

Treatment

Abstinence is essential; nutritional support; glucocorticoids are probably beneficial for treatment of severe disease.

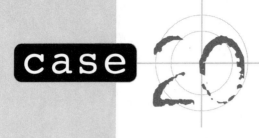

case 20

ID/CC A 65-year-old **alcoholic man** presents with right upper quadrant pain, **jaundice, anorexia,** and progressive **abdominal distention** of 2-month duration; the distention has rapidly worsened over the past 10 days.

HPI He also complains of **weight loss.** He has a **history of chronic hepatitis** but has no history of hematemesis, melena, hematochezia, or altered sensorium.

PE Jaundice; **palmar erythema; spider angiomata** over upper abdomen; **loss of axillary and pubic hair; nodular hepatomegaly; free fluid in peritoneal cavity** (ASCITES); mildly enlarged spleen.

Labs Increased direct bilirubin; **decreased serum albumin;** increased serum transaminase; mildly elevated alkaline phosphatase; **prolonged PT; markedly elevated serum α-fetoprotein (AFP);** positive serum hepatitis B virus (HBsAg) surface antigen.

Imaging US/CT/MR: irregular **hepatic mass** that appears as a high-intensity pattern on T2-weighted images and a low-intensity pattern on T1-weighted images; enlarged spleen; **enlarged portal vein; ascites.**

case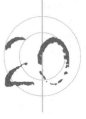

Hepatocellular Carcinoma

Differential

Cholangiocarcinoma

Hepatic adenoma

Hemangioma

Metastatic disease

Discussion

Hepatocellular carcinoma is a malignant primary neoplasm of the liver. In the Western world, it **usually arises from a cirrhotic liver** and, wherever prevalent, is frequently associated with **hepatitis B** and hepatitis C infection. Other predisposing conditions include hemochromatosis, Wilson disease, α_1-antitrypsin deficiency, alcoholic cirrhosis, and aflatoxin B1. It is spread by **hematogenous** and lymphatic dissemination, often to the lungs.

Treatment

Surgical resection and transplantation in resectable cases; other therapies that may be employed include chemoembolization, radiofrequency ablation, radiotherapy, and systemic chemotherapy.

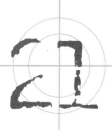

case 21

ID/CC A 50-year-old man with advanced **alcoholic cirrhosis** develops **oliguria** and **abdominal distention**.

HPI His **renal and electrolyte status** has been **steadily deteriorating**.

PE VS: tachycardia. PE: jaundice; ascites; asterixis.

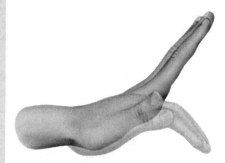

Figure 21-1. The flapping tremor of asterixis.

Labs Low GFR (creatinine level >1.5 mg/dL or 24-hour creatinine clearance <40 mL/min); low urinary sodium excretion (<5 mEq/L); urine osmolality greater than plasma osmolality; serum sodium concentration <130 mEq/L. UA: no active sediment.

Gross Pathology Renal biopsy shows no abnormality.

case 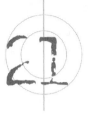 21

Hepatorenal Syndrome

Differential

Acute tubular necrosis

Acute glomerulonephritis

Prerenal azotemia

Drug-induced nephropathy

Treatment

Reversal of renal failure can occur with successful liver transplantation. In contrast, survival on dialysis is generally limited by the severity of the hepatic failure. No proven drug therapy.

Discussion

Hepatorenal syndrome (HRS) refers to the development of acute renal failure in a patient with advanced hepatic disease. It is often caused by **fulminant hepatic failure, cirrhosis,** and, less frequently, by a **metastatic tumor** or **severe alcoholic hepatitis.** HRS usually represents the end stage of a **reduction in renal perfusion** induced by increasingly severe hepatic injury. It carries a **high mortality.**

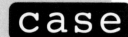 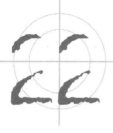

ID/CC A 65-year-old man with **unresectable carcinoma of the sigmoid colon** is evaluated for **hepatomegaly** that was detected on a follow-up exam.

HPI The patient is undergoing chemotherapy and underwent palliative surgery 1 month ago.

PE Marked **pallor; large nodular liver palpable;** ascites (due to peritoneal seeding); colostomy bag noted.

Labs **Markedly elevated carcinoembryonic antigen (CEA)** levels; **markedly raised alkaline phosphatase;** other LFTs normal.

Imaging CT/US, abdomen: multiple enhancing hepatic nodules. Sigmoidoscopy: infiltrating **"napkin-ring"** growth in sigmoid colon.

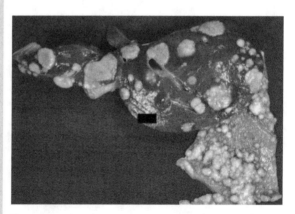

Figure 22-1. Multiple discrete, white, irregularly shaped masses in the liver.

Gross Pathology On autopsy, multiple nodules noted, some with central necrosis (due to insufficient vascular supply).

case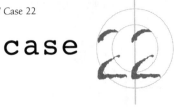

Metastatic Carcinoma—Liver

Differential

Cavernous hemangioma
Cholangiocarcinoma
Focal nodular hyperplasia
Extramedullary hematopoiesis

Discussion

Liver metastases are more common than primary tumors of the liver. The most common tumors that metastasize to the liver are colon, gastric, pancreatic, breast, and lung carcinomas.

Treatment

Supportive management; consider radiofrequency ablation for solitary metastasis.

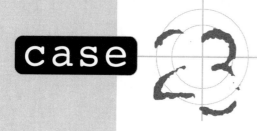

case

ID/CC A 34-year-old **alcoholic** man complains of sudden-onset, unrelenting **midepigastric pain radiating to the lower thoracic spine.**

HPI He also complains of associated **anorexia, nausea,** and **vomiting.** The pain becomes worse when he is supine.

PE VS: **hypotension; tachycardia.** PE: pale, sweaty; in severe distress; **periumbilical ecchymoses** (CULLEN SIGN); **left flank ecchymosis** (GREY TURNER SIGN); marked **epigastric tenderness** and diffuse **rebound tenderness** but minimal rigidity; abdomen distended with markedly decreased bowel sounds.

Labs CBC: leukocytosis. **Markedly elevated serum amylase** and **lipase; elevated glucose;** elevated SGOT and LDH; **hypocalcemia.** ABGs: hypoxemia.

Imaging CXR/KUB: no free air under diaphragm; abrupt termination of gaseous transverse colon at splenic flexure (COLON CUTOFF SIGN); distended loop of bowel in proximal jejunum (SENTINEL LOOP). CT, abdomen: enlargement and **inhomogeneity** of pancreas; **streaky peripancreatic inflammation** and fluid collection.

Gross Pathology Autopsy: pancreas reveals pasty white foci of **fat necrosis, hemorrhage,** and cystic cavitation.

Micro Pathology Edema of connective tissue, polymorphonuclear infiltration, hemorrhage and necrosis of pancreatic acini; fat necrosis appears as pale blue amorphous foci where adipocyte membranes are dissolved.

case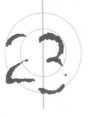

Pancreatitis—Acute

Differential

Abdominal aneurysm

Cholelithiasis

Gastroenteritis

Hepatitis

Small bowel obstruction

Discussion

Gallstones and **alcohol abuse** are etiologic factors in 90% of patients with acute pancreatitis. Gallstones are thought to cause pancreatitis by **transient obstruction at the ampulla of Vater,** which leads to increased pancreatic ductal pressure. Other causes include infections (e.g., mumps), hereditary pancreatitis, shock, acute ischemia, hypercalcemia, hypertriglyceridemia, and drugs (e.g., thiazides, sulfonamides). Complications include DIC, **shock,** ARDS, hypocalcemia, acute renal failure, and pancreatic pseudocyst. Prognosis can be determined empirically by the Ranson criteria.

▩ TABLE 23-1 POOR PROGNOSTIC FEATURES IN PANCREATITIS

At admission
  Age >55
  WBC count >16,000
  Glucose >200 mg/100 mL
  LDH >350
  AST >250
During 48 hours after admission
  Hct >10-point decrease
  BUN >5 mg/100 mL increase
  Ca^{2+} <8.0
  pO_2 <60 mm Hg on room air
  Base excess >4 mEq/L
  Estimated fluid sequestration >6,000 mL

AST, aspartate aminotransferase; BUN, blood urea nitrogen; Hct, hematocrit; LDH, lactate dehydrogenase; WBC, white blood cell.

Treatment

"Rest" the pancreas (analgesics, IV fluids, no oral intake, parenteral nutrition, nasogastric suction); cessation of alcohol use.

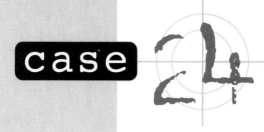

case 24

ID/CC A 24-year-old white woman complains of **crampy abdominal pain,** inability to pass flatus, abdominal distention, nausea, and vomiting.

HPI After lack of improvement with 24 hours of nasogastric-tube suction and IV fluid, she underwent laparotomy to relieve **bowel obstruction** (due to a large hamartoma).

PE **Hyperpigmented macules** on **lips** and **buccal mucosa** and on palms, fingers, and toes; **multiple hamartomatous growths** palpated **throughout GI tract.**

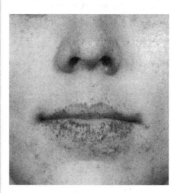

Figure 24-1. Perioral melanin pigmentation.

Labs CBC/PBS: **microcytic, hypochromic anemia** (due to moderate GI bleeding). **Positive stool guaiac** test.

Imaging UGI/SBFT/BE: acute small bowel obstruction; multiple **polypoid growths** of jejunum, ileum, and colon.

Gross Pathology Pedunculated nodules up to 2 cm in size in stomach, duodenum, jejunum, ileum, and colon.

Micro Pathology **Increased melanin deposition in buccal mucosa and lips;** hamartomatous lesions rarely undergo malignant transformation; smooth muscle and connective tissue extend into the pedunculated polyps and form an arborizing network.

case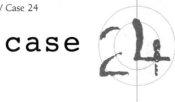

Peutz–Jeghers Syndrome

Differential
Familial adenomatous polyposis
Cowden disease
Juvenile polyposis syndrome
Neurofibromatosis

Discussion
Peutz–Jeghers syndrome is **autosomal dominant** and is one type of hereditary familial polyposis syndrome. Polyps are hamartomas with **low malignant potential,** so resection is performed only if polyps are symptomatic. The condition is associated with an **increased risk of extra-intestinal cancer** (e.g., pancreas, breast, lung, ovary, uterus).

Treatment
Periodic surveillance; consider endoscopic removal of hemorrhagic or large (>5 mm) polyps; treat complications such as **obstruction, intussusception, and bleeding.**

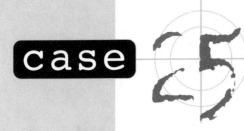

case

ID/CC   A **50-year-old** white **woman** complains of dizziness, fatigue, weight loss, and **difficulty swallowing** solid food (DYSPHAGIA).

HPI   She has been concerned about a recent **craving for ice and clay** (PICA). She reports no nausea/vomiting or hematemesis/melena.

PE   VS: tachycardia. PE: pale skin and mucous membranes; **spoon-shaped nails** (KOILONYCHIA); **smooth, shiny red tongue** (GLOSSITIS); stomatitis.

Labs   CBC/PBS: **microcytic, hypochromic anemia. Low serum iron.**

Imaging   UGI: thin membranes of squamous mucosa typically in mid- or upper esophagus (ESOPHAGEAL WEBBING).

Gross Pathology   Postcricoid esophageal concentric web.

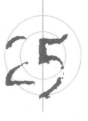

case 25

Plummer–Vinson Syndrome

Differential

Achalasia

Esophageal stricture

Esophageal cancer

Stricture

Discussion

Also called Paterson–Kelly syndrome, Plummer–Vinson syndrome is associated with an **increased risk of esophageal cancer**. However, it is not a malignant condition in itself.

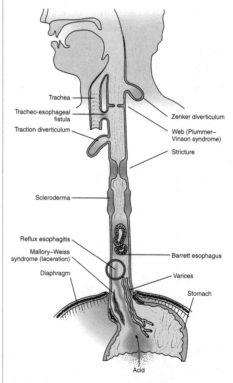

Figure 25-1. Summary of non-neoplastic esophageal conditions.

Treatment

Esophageal dilatation; supplemental iron; investigate and treat cause of iron deficiency anemia.

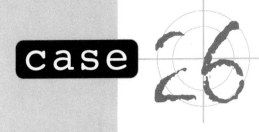

case 26

ID/CC   A 55-year-old **woman** presents with increasing yellowing of the eyes (JAUNDICE), fatigue, and **chronic itching.**

HPI   She also has **rheumatoid arthritis and chronic thyroiditis.** She has no prior history of jaundice, does not drink alcohol, and has never received a blood transfusion.

PE   **Icterus;** numerous scratch marks and excoriations on the skin; xanthomas and **xanthelasma;** hepatomegaly, splenomegaly, and no ascites; rheumatoid joint deformities and goiter (due to chronic thyroiditis).

Labs   Raised ESR; **markedly elevated alkaline phosphatase;** elevated serum IgM levels; mildly elevated direct bilirubin and aminotransferases; **elevated serum cholesterol** (>300 mg/dL); high titers of serum **antimitochondrial antibody;** diagnostic liver biopsy.

Gross Pathology   Dark green, enlarged liver.

Micro Pathology   Bile duct destruction with lymphocytic-plasmacytic infiltration of portal areas; **periportal epithelioid granuloma formation** and portal scarring with linking of portal tracts; periportal bile stasis noted.

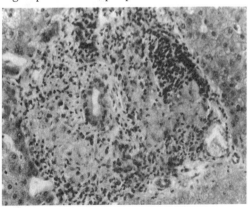

Figure 26-1. Lymphocytic infiltration with granuloma formation around the portal area.

51

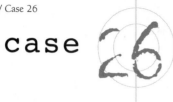

case

Primary Biliary Cirrhosis

Differential

Autoimmune hepatitis
Biliary obstruction
Sarcoidosis
Primary sclerosing cholangitis
Graft vs. host disease

Discussion

Primary biliary cirrhosis is a chronic liver disease of probable **autoimmune** etiology that occurs primarily in **middle-aged women** and is characterized by **non-suppurative obliterative cholangitis that progresses to cirrhosis**; it is associated with other autoimmune diseases in 85% of cases. Complications include cirrhosis and portal hypertension, malabsorption due to steatorrhea, and osteoporosis due to malabsorption of vitamin D and calcium.

Treatment

Cholestyramine to control pruritus; ursodeoxycholic acid (UDCA); immunosuppression; liver transplantation is the only definitive treatment.

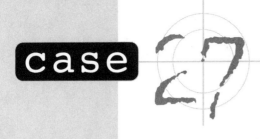

case 27

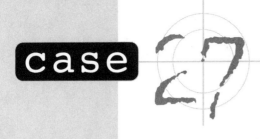

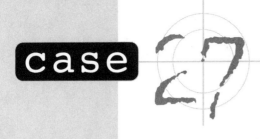

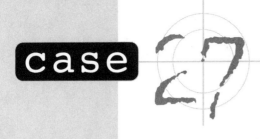

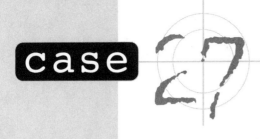

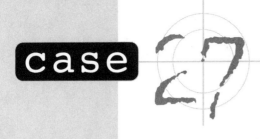

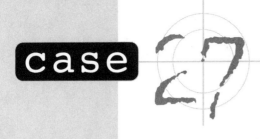

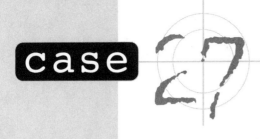

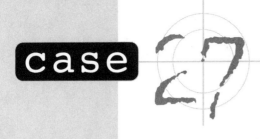

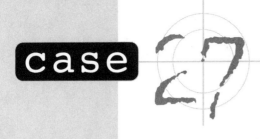

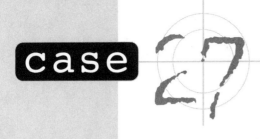

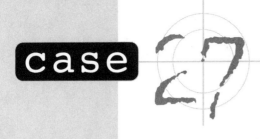

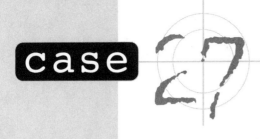

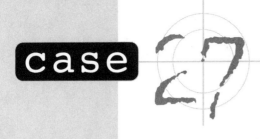

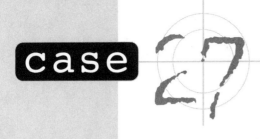

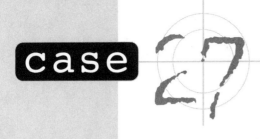

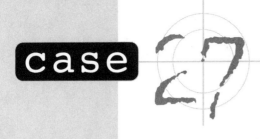

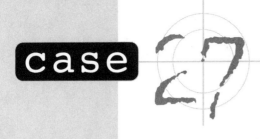

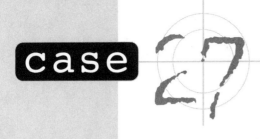

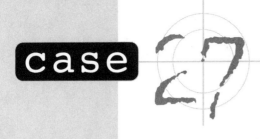

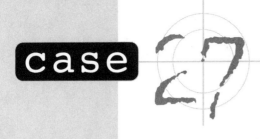

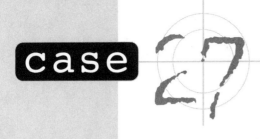

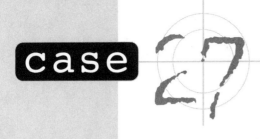

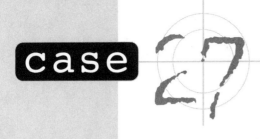

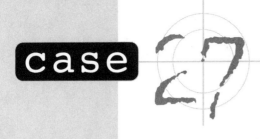

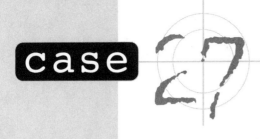

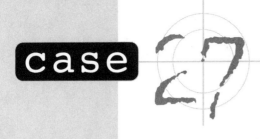

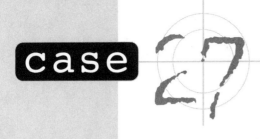

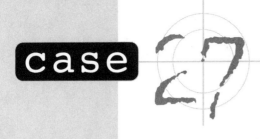

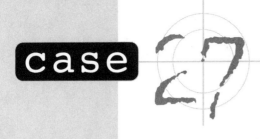

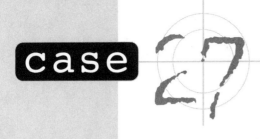

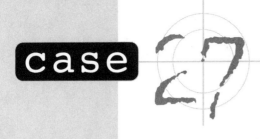

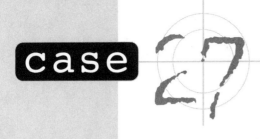

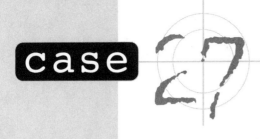

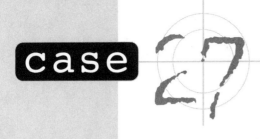

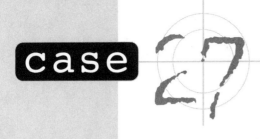

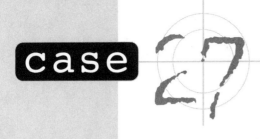

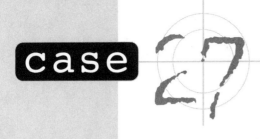

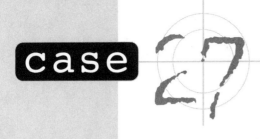

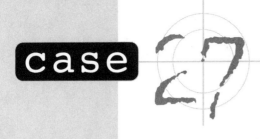

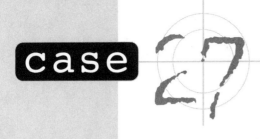

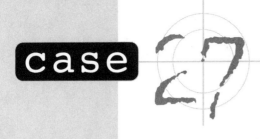

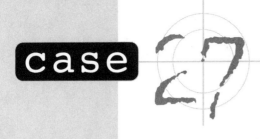

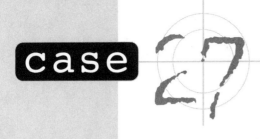

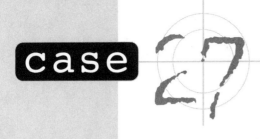

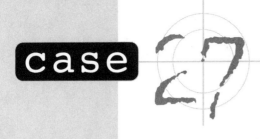

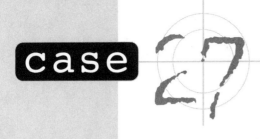

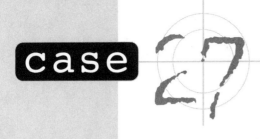

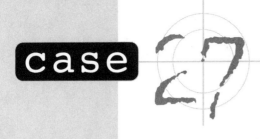

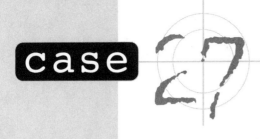

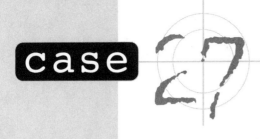

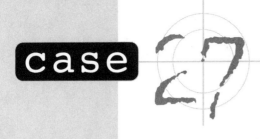

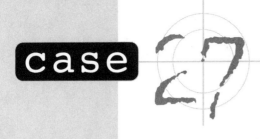

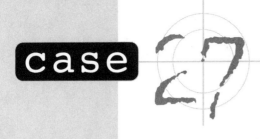

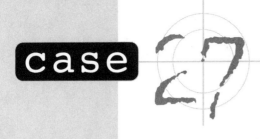

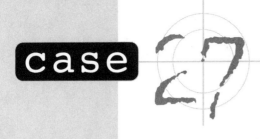

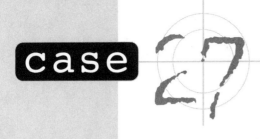

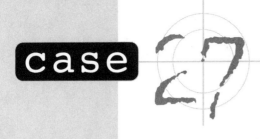

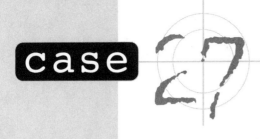

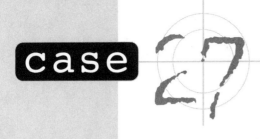

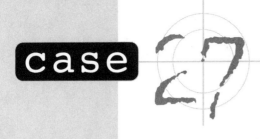

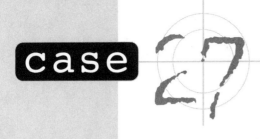

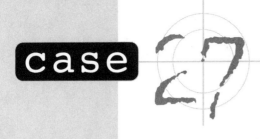

case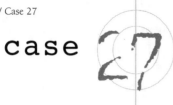

Protocolitis

Differential

Ulcerative colitis

Infectious colitis (see below)

Infectious diarrhea

Radiation changes

Discussion

The term **"gay bowel syndrome"** is used in reference to enteric and perirectal infections that are commonly encountered in immune-competent homosexual men; in homosexuals with HIV, opportunistic organisms play a more important role. Common etiologic agents include *Chlamydia trachomatis*, lymphogranuloma venereum serovars, *Neisseria gonorrhoeae*, HSV, *Treponema pallidum*, human papillomavirus, *Campylobacter* species, *Shigella*, *Entamoeba histolytica*, and *Giardia*.

Treatment

Ceftriaxone and **doxycycline** (to treat likely concomitant chlamydial infection) for both patient and partner. Most apparent failures of correct antibiotic therapy are in fact due to reinfection; in resistant cases, **spectinomycin, fluoroquinolones,** or other **cephalosporins** can be used.

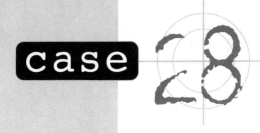

ID/CC A 25-year-old man, a U.S. citizen on **vacation in Mexico,** presents with abrupt-onset explosive **watery diarrhea, abdominal cramps,** and a **low-grade fever** and chills.

HPI The patient does not complain of tenesmus or passage of blood or mucus in his stools, but he does complain of a feeling of **urgency** to defecate.

PE VS: low-grade fever. PE: unremarkable.

Labs No erythrocytes, WBCs, or parasites seen in stained stool; bioassays for enterotoxigenic *Escherichia coli* **(ETEC)** reveal presence of the labile **enterotoxin (LT)** (tests available only for research purposes).

case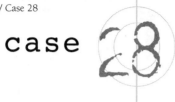

Traveler's Diarrhea

Differential

Viral gastroenteritis

Bacterial gastroenteritis (see below)

Crohn disease

Protozoal gastroenteritis

Meckel diverticula

Colon cancer

Discussion

Traveler's diarrhea is a self-limited condition that develops within 1 to 2 days of ingestion of contaminated food or drinks. Greater than three-fourths of cases of traveler's diarrhea are caused by bacteria, with enterotoxigenic *E. coli* the most frequent cause (may also be caused by enteropathogenic *E. coli* and, in Mexico, by an enteroadherent *E. coli*). Other common pathogens include *Shigella* species, *Campylobacter jejuni, Aeromonas* species, *Plesiomonas shigelloides, Salmonella* species, and noncholera vibrios. Rotavirus and Norwalk agent are the most common viral causes; *Giardia, Cryptosporidium,* and, rarely, *Entamoeba histolytica* are parasitic pathogens. Enterotoxigenic *E. coli* produce enterotoxins that bind to intestinal receptors and **activate adenyl cyclase** in the intestinal cell to produce an increase in the level of the cyclic nucleotides cAMP (LT, labile toxin) and cGMP (ST, stable toxin), which markedly augments sodium, chloride, and water loss, thereby producing a **secretory diarrhea.**

Treatment

Fluid replacement; antibiotics (fluoroquinolone or TMP-SMX) with loperamide; prevention with careful hygienic practices and prophylactic fluoroquinolone or bismuth subsalicylate with loperamide.

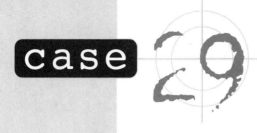

ID/CC A 60-year-old man presents with complaints of **fever, generalized abdominal pain, persistent bloody diarrhea, and increasing rectal pain.**

HPI He was diagnosed with ulcerative colitis several years ago and had been treated with sulfasalazine and prednisone for intermittent exacerbations.

PE VS: fever (39.9°C); tachycardia (HR 120); mild hypotension (BP 88/50). PE: **toxic-looking patient;** pallor noted; abdominal exam reveals **generalized tenderness** and **reduced bowel sounds.**

Labs CBC: normocytic, normochromic anemia. RBCs, pus, and epithelial cells seen on stool exam.

Imaging XR, abdomen (including cross-table lateral): colonic dilation measuring >6 cm in diameter; **moderate dilatation** of **descending colon; thickened colonic wall** (due to wall edema); loss of colonic haustrations.

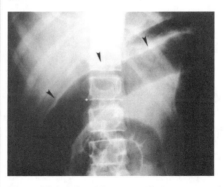

Figure 29-1. Dilated but smooth transverse colon with no haustral markings (arrows).

Gross Pathology Moderate dilatation of colon; rectal mucosa friable and swollen; complete loss of mucosal folds.

Micro Pathology Diffuse mononuclear infiltrate in lamina propria with neutrophils, mast cells, and eosinophils.

57

case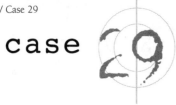

Toxic Megacolon

Differential

Crohn disease

Cytomegalovirus colitis

Pseudomembranous colitis

Ulcerative colitis

Hirschsprung disease

Chagas disease

Discussion

Toxic megacolon results from complete shutdown of colonic neuromuscular function due to inflammation of the **myenteric neural plexus**. It may be seen as a complication of Crohn disease, **ischemic colitis, pseudomembranous colitis,** and **ulcerative colitis.**

Treatment

Bowel decompression with nasogastric suction; fluid and electrolyte replacement; **parenteral antibiotics** to prevent sepsis; corticosteroids may be indicated to suppress inflammatory reaction in gut; **surgical colectomy** if immediate medical measures fail.

case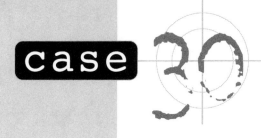

ID/CC A 31-year-old man complains of having more than five bowel movements a day together with **cramping abdominal pain** and **tenesmus**.

HPI The patient adds that his stools consist of watery or pasty material with **mucus** and gross quantities of **blood**. He also complains of intermittent fatigue, fever, and an increased need for sleep.

PE VS: mild fever. PE: localized tenderness over distal colon.

Labs CBC: anemia; leukocytosis; hypoalbuminemia. Elevated ESR; stool exam reveals **no parasites; no bacterial pathogen** isolated in culture. P-ANCA positive; ASCA negative.

Imaging BE: early mucosal granularity; later, rigidity and **loss of haustrations** ("LEAD PIPE"), with ragged ulcerated mucosa and ulcerations. Colonoscopy: **mucosal erythema and granularity** with hemorrhaging and **inflammatory pseudopolyps.**

Gross Pathology Scarring and coarse, granular mucosal surface indicating presence of microulcerations; mucosal surface is friable; **lesions are continuous** from anal to oral direction.

Micro Pathology Increased numbers of lymphocytes, plasma cells, and PMNs; atrophy of mucosal glands and presence of PMNs in crypts of Lieberkühn (often called crypt abscesses); inflammatory changes confined to mucosa and submucosa.

case

Ulcerative Colitis

Differential | Pseudomembranous colitis
Crohn disease
Colon cancer
Rectal carcinoma

Discussion | Patients with ulcerative colitis are at **increased risk for colon cancer.** Factors favoring the development of colon cancer in ulcerative colitis are the duration of disease for 8 years or longer, involvement of the entire colon, continuous clinical activity, and, possibly, a severe initial attack. It is routinely advised that patients undergo regular surveillance that includes colonoscopy and an examination of multiple biopsies for dysplastic changes or frank cancer. Major complications include toxic megacolon and massive intestinal hemorrhage with shock and sepsis. Extra-intestinal manifestations may include arthritis, erythema nodosum, ankylosing spondylitis, and sclerosing cholangitis.

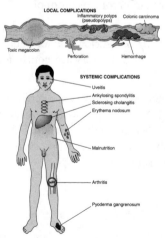

Figure 30-1. Complications of ulcerative colitis.

Treatment | Sulfasalazine, 5-ASA preparations; glucocorticoids; cyclosporine for severe colitis; surgery if indicated (total proctocolectomy is curative).

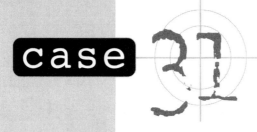

ID/CC	A 56-year-old white man complains of **diarrhea** and bloating for **several months** along with ankle swelling.
HPI	He also complains of memory loss, fever, **arthritis** in the knees and hands, and **weight loss.**
PE	VS: fever. PE: thin, gaunt man; muscle wasting; swollen, tender right wrist and ankle; axillary and femoral lymphadenopathy; ecchymoses of chest and arms.
Labs	CBC/PBS: macrocytic, hypochromic anemia; hypoalbuminemia; **increased fecal fat** (steatorrhea). *Tropheryma whippelii* DNA detected on **PCR.**
Imaging	UGI/SBFT: nonspecific dilatation of small bowel.
Gross Pathology	Atrophy of intestinal mucosa; inflammatory infiltrate in synovia of joints.
Micro Pathology	Small bowel biopsy reveals **characteristic macrophages** containing bacilli with **periodic acid-Schiff (PAS)** reagent staining; characteristic gram-negative actinomycete bacilli in macrophages, PMNs, and epithelial cells of lamina propria; dilated lymphatics; flattening of intestinal villi.

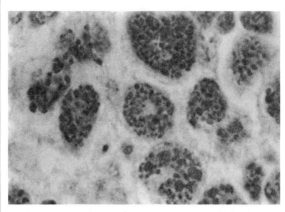

Figure 31-1. PAS-stained inclusions within macrophages of the intestinal mucosa.

case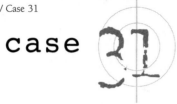

Whipple Disease

Differential

Ischemic bowel disease
Celiac sprue
Mycobacterium avium intracellular
Abetalipoproteinemia
AIDS-related complex

Discussion

Caused by infection with *T. whippelii*; produces **malabsorption** of fat-soluble vitamins, protein, iron, folic acid, and vitamin B_{12}.

Treatment

Bactrim (TMP-SMX), penicillin, or amoxicillin for several months to a year or until infection is eradicated.

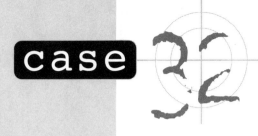

case 32

ID/CC	A 43-year-old white man complains of severe **burning epigastric pain** and **diarrhea** of 2-year duration that has been refractory to medical management.
HPI	The pain awakens him early in the morning, is accompanied by nausea and vomiting, increases with coffee consumption, and also appears 2 to 3 hours after meals. Three days ago, he also noticed **black stools.**
PE	Slight discomfort on epigastric palpation but no signs of peritoneal irritation; pale skin and mucous membranes; **occult blood** on digital rectal exam.
Labs	Fasting **serum gastrin markedly increased; increased gastric acid output** (HYPERCHLORHYDRIA) (due to elevated gastrin).
Imaging	CT/MR/Angio: small lesion in pancreas, difficult to localize. UGI/SBFT: atypical ulcers; gastric fold thickening.
Gross Pathology	**Ulcers in uncommon places** in esophagus, duodenum, and jejunum (due to excessive gastrin secretion); **gastrinoma** (commonly in pancreas or duodenum).
Micro Pathology	Usually originate from **delta cells** of pancreas; original lesion may be adenoma, hyperplasia, or carcinoma; hyperplasia of antral gastrin-producing cells.

case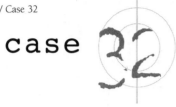

Zollinger–Ellison Syndrome

Differential	Retained gastric antrum
	G-cell hyperplasia
	Gastric outlet obstruction
	Small bowel obstruction
Discussion	Zollinger–Ellison syndrome causes painful chronic diarrhea (vs. intestinal parasites, carcinoid syndrome, ulcerative colitis); roughly half may be malignant. It is associated with **multiple endocrine neoplasia (MEN) type I** (WERMER SYNDROME).
Treatment	High-dose proton pump inhibitors (omeprazole, lansoprazole); surgical resection if well localized and no metastases; gastrectomy; vagotomy.

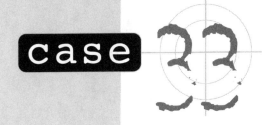

case 32

ID/CC A 32-year-old homeless white man is brought to the emergency room by an ambulance following **convulsions** that took place on the street.

HPI The patient is disheveled and unshaven in his appearance. A history cannot be obtained because he is alone and unable to respond to questions.

PE Dehydration; **jaundice; alcohol on breath;** 2-cm laceration on occipital area with no bleeding; semicomatose state with response to pain only; pupils equal; **fine tremor** in extremities; palmar erythema; **hepatomegaly.**

Labs CBC/PBS: **macrocytic, hypochromic anemia.** **Elevated** direct and indirect **bilirubin; elevated AST and ALT;** AST/ALT ratio of 2:1; **elevated alkaline phosphatase; elevated PT; low serum albumin;** hypoglycemia.

Gross Pathology **Fatty liver;** micronodular **cirrhosis;** marked **gastritis;** bronchial aspiration.

Micro Pathology Hepatocytes distended with fat; hepatocellular necrosis; **Mallory bodies** (hyaline); cytoplasmic vacuolization of stem cells in bone marrow; myofibrillar necrosis; diffuse axonal degeneration.

case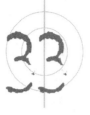

Alcoholism

Differential

Anxiety disorder
Bipolar disorder
Depression
Panic disorder
Drug abuse

Discussion

Alcoholic delirium tremens (**DT**s) usually occur 2 to 5 days after cessation of drinking and are characterized by seizures, delusions, agitation, disorientation, visual and tactile hallucinations, and autonomic instability. DT prophylaxis consists of benzodiazepines and restraints to prevent damage to patient and to others. DTs have a mortality rate of 15% if untreated.

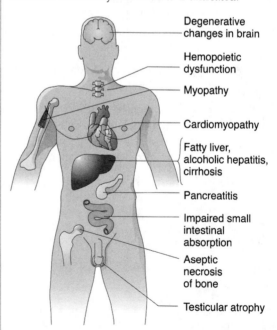

Figure 33-1. Complications of chronic alcohol abuse.

Treatment

Vitamins (thiamine and folate); glucose; rehydration; treat acute withdrawal and DTs with benzodiazepines.

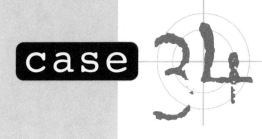

ID/CC A 49-year-old **man**, an immigrant who is a native of Guam, has seen three doctors in his country and tried different therapies for marked, **progressive weakness** of his hands and arms, **difficulty speaking**, muscle wasting in both hands, and troublesome **involuntary muscle contractions** (FASCICULATIONS).

HPI He has no history of sensory symptoms, bladder or bowel dysfunction, fever, exanthem, dog bites, vaccinations, or spinal or cranial trauma.

PE Lower motor neuron signs: **bilateral wasting of hands**, deep tendon reflexes absent in upper limbs, **muscle weakness, fasciculations**; upper motor neuron signs: positive Babinski sign, stiffness and spasticity of upper limbs; normal fundus, sensory system, and cranial nerves.

Labs LP: **CSF normal. Slightly elevated CK**; normal TSH, T_3, and T_4 levels; normal serum calcium and glucose. EMG: diffuse denervation, normal conduction velocity, and decreased amplitude of compound muscle action potentials.

Imaging CT/MR, brain: **brain normal.**

Micro Pathology Nonspecific atrophy on muscle biopsy.

NEUROLOGY

67

case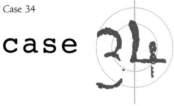

Amyotrophic Lateral Sclerosis

Differential

Brain stem glioma

Chronic inflammatory demyelinating polyneuropathy

Myasthenia gravis

Leptomeningeal carcinomatosis

Neurosarcoidosis

Spinal muscle atrophy

Discussion

Also known as **Lou Gehrig disease,** amyotrophic lateral sclerosis (ALS) is a slowly progressive, generalized motor muscle paralysis involving both upper and lower motor neurons. Death ultimately occurs as a result of respiratory insufficiency secondary to muscle weakness. Patients often have multiple respiratory infections, secondary to aspiration. Deterioration to a bedridden state predisposes to decubitus ulcers and skin infections. Nearly 10% of cases are familial and transmitted in an autosomal dominant fashion. The most common mutations in such cases are in the gene for the enzyme superoxide dismutase (SOD). This offers some insight into the pathology of the disorder, with oxidative damage to neurons playing a central role.

Treatment

Largely supportive; disease is progressive and fatal.

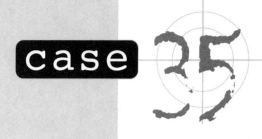

case 25

ID/CC   A **60-year-old** man presents with **speech difficulties**.

HPI   The patient developed this difficulty following a **left-sided stroke** from which he is currently recovering. He has **diabetes** and has been on insulin for 10 years; he is also a **chronic smoker.**

PE   Speech **lacks fluency;** patient has difficulty **finding certain words** and sometimes **produces wrong word; comprehension is well preserved,** as are higher mental functions; ability to repeat is better than spontaneous speech; associated recovering right-sided aphasia noted; motor weakness of right upper and lower limbs with exaggerated deep tendon reflexes and right-sided Babinski reflex.

Labs   Elevated blood glucose; remainder of tests normal.

Imaging CT: **infarct in region of left frontoparietal cortex.**

case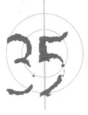

Aphasia—Broca Area

Differential

Developmental disorder

Mutism

Psychiatric disease

Head injury

Dementia

Intracranial neoplasm

Discussion

This patient has Broca dysphasia (expressive, nonfluent) with an associated right hemiplegia. The brain damage causing this condition is believed to involve the **dominant inferior frontal gyrus** (BROCA AREA). In contrast to patients with Wernicke aphasia, patients with Broca aphasia have insight into their condition and are thus at high risk for depression.

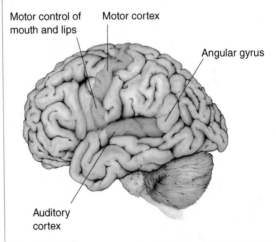

Figure 35-1. Key components of the language system in the left hemisphere.

Treatment

Speech therapy in addition to physiotherapy for stroke; long-term low-dose **aspirin**.

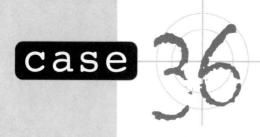
ID/CC A 20-year-old man is brought to the ER after falling from a ladder.

HPI He fell vertically so that his head hit the ground first. Despite the injury, he is conscious and **does not report any neurologic deficit,** only severe pain in his neck.

PE **No neurologic deficit found** on clinical examination.

Imaging XR, cervical spine: **burst fracture of atlas.** CT, cervical spine: rules out C1–C2 instability and associated injuries.

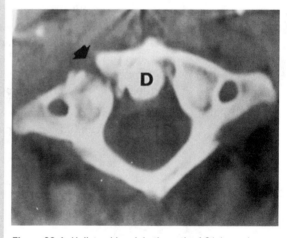

Figure 36-1. Unilateral break in the arch of C1 (arrow).

NEUROLOGY

71

case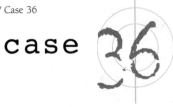

C1 Spinal Cord Injury

Differential

Cervical strain
Vertebral artery dissection
Spinal cord infection
Spinal cord neoplasm
Torticollis
Thoracic outlet syndrome

Discussion

The most common mechanism of injury in patients with Jefferson fracture is axial loading. Other cervical spine injuries include **atlantoaxial fracture dislocation,** more frequently associated with neurologic deficit; displacement is commonly anterior, and treatment consists of **skull traction** followed by **immobilization.** A **violent flexion–compression** force may result in a **sudden prolapse of the nucleus pulposus** of the cervical disk into the vertebral canal, producing quadriplegia; here an **early decompression** is required.

Treatment

Inherently unstable fracture requiring halo jacket immobilization and fusion if nonunion occurs.

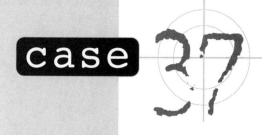

case 27

ID/CC A **70-year-old man** presents with dull, aching **pain in both calves after moderate exercise.**

HPI The symptoms started a few months ago, typically developing after the patient walked 300 to 400 yards; **symptoms were relieved after a few minutes' rest or when the patient sat down and stooped forward** (pseudoclaudication). In addition to the pain, the patient has experienced numbness in his thighs. He has had no sphincter disturbance but has had **low back pain for many years.**

PE Spinal exam reveals **loss of lumbar lordosis** and reduced flexion and extension of lumbar spine; tone, power, and coordination in lower limbs normal; **reflexes in lower limbs symmetrical but reduced compared to upper limbs**; plantar reflexes flexor; peripheral arterial pulses **present** both at rest and after exercise.

Labs Lab parameters normal.

Imaging XR, lumbar spine: lumbar spondylosis with marked osteophyte formation. CT, spine: **lumbar spinal canal stenosis confirmed.**

case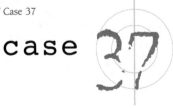

Cauda Equina Syndrome

Differential

Cervical strain
Vertebral artery dissection
Spinal cord infection
Spinal cord neoplasm
Torticollis
Thoracic outlet syndrome

Discussion

A number of mechanisms may lead to lumbar canal stenosis, including osteoarthritis with hypertrophy of the facet joints, disk prolapse, surgery, spondylolisthesis, Paget disease, neoplasia, and infection; any of these conditions may be superimposed on a congenitally narrow spinal canal. The anteroposterior diameter of the cord is narrowed during extension, which tends to compromise the blood supply of the cord, resulting in the development of symptoms; stooping forward does the reverse and therefore relieves symptoms.

Treatment

Surgery requiring laminectomy at various levels.

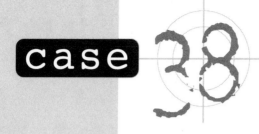

ID/CC A 40-year-old man complains of the **"worst headache of his life"** and **double vision**.

HPI He has been **projectile vomiting**. He has no history of fever or neck stiffness.

PE **Papilledema on funduscopic exam; right eye deviated laterally and downward** (due to right third cranial nerve palsy); other cranial nerves normal; no meningeal signs noted; motor system examination normal.

Labs Routine laboratory tests normal.

Imaging Angio, cerebral: posterior communicating (PCOM) artery aneurysm. CT, head: enhancing mass impinging over right third nerve.

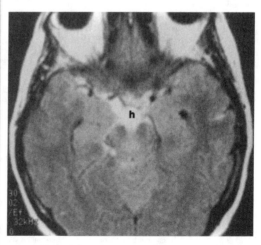

Figure 38-1. Subarachnoid hemorrhage(h) in the basilar cisterns.

case 38

Cerebral Aneurysm

Differential
Cervical strain
Vertebral artery dissection
Spinal cord infection
Spinal cord neoplasm
Torticollis
Thoracic outlet syndrome

Discussion
Congenital berry aneurysms are associated with **polycystic kidney disease** and **arteriovenous malformation;** they may rupture (during sexual activity, weightlifting, straining) and cause **subarachnoid hemorrhage.**

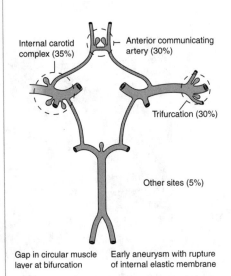

Internal carotid complex (35%)

Anterior communicating artery (30%)

Trifurcation (30%)

Other sites (5%)

Gap in circular muscle layer at bifurcation

Early aneurysm with rupture of internal elastic membrane

Figure 38-2. Common locations of berry aneurysms.

Treatment
Endovascular or neurosurgical clipping of aneurysm.

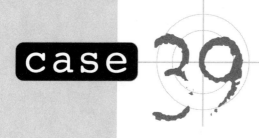

ID/CC A 14-year-old white **boy** comes into the emergency room because of **projectile vomiting** and a severe **headache**.

HPI He has a history of unexplained **short stature** and **polyuria**.

PE **Papilledema and optic disk swelling** (due to increased intracranial pressure) on funduscopic exam; confusion; visual field testing reveals **bitemporal hemianopia**; no other focal neurologic signs; no neurocutaneous markers or meningeal signs.

Imaging XR, skull: **enlarged sella turcica.** CT/MR: **enhancing**, cystic, multilobulated **suprasellar mass with ring calcification**; hydrocephalus (due to obstruction of foramen of Monro and aqueduct of Sylvius).

NEUROLOGY

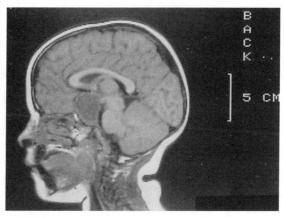

Figure 39-1. A large suprasellar mass.

Gross Pathology Cystic mass with concentric areas of calcification.

Micro Pathology Mixture of squamous epithelial elements and delicate reticular stroma; gliosis seen at periphery; cholesterol-rich cystic fluid.

77

case 39

Craniopharyngioma

Differential

Astrocytoma

Ependymoma

Neuroblastoma

Primitive neuroectoderm tumor

Pituitary adenoma

Discussion

Craniopharyngioma is the **most common supratentorial brain tumor in children** and is embryologically derived from **Rathke pouch remnants.** It is a common cause of growth retardation, diabetes insipidus (compression of pituitary), bitemporal hemianopia (compression of optic chiasm), and headache (obstructive hydrocephalus). It shows a bimodal age distribution with a second peak in the fifth decade.

Treatment

Surgical removal; radiotherapy.

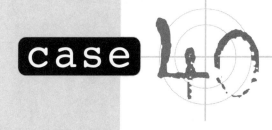

ID/CC	A 62-year-old man is brought to his family doctor because of rapidly progressive loss of cognitive function (DEMENTIA) and excessive **somnolence.**
HPI	About 5 years ago, he received a **corneal transplant.** His wife states that she has seen a definite **change in his personality** over the past year.
PE	**Dementia; myoclonic fasciculations;** normal funduscopic exam; no other focal neurologic signs.
Labs	LP: **normal CSF profile.** EEG: bursts of high-voltage slow-wave activity and slow background.
Imaging	CT, head: ventricular enlargement and cerebral atrophy. MR, brain: increased signal intensity in affected areas. PET, brain: areas of diminished glucose metabolism.
Micro Pathology	Brain biopsy shows amyloid deposition, **spongiform degeneration,** decrease in neurons of cerebral cortex, and astrocytic proliferation; no inflammatory changes seen.

NEUROLOGY

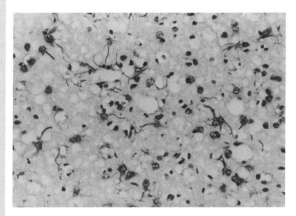

Figure 40-1. Spongiosis of the neuropil.

case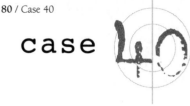

Creutzfeldt–Jakob Disease

Differential

Alzheimer disease

Herpes simplex encephalitis

Hydrocephalus

Multi-infarct dementia

Thyroid disease

Vitamin B_{12} deficiency

Discussion

A **subacute spongiform encephalopathy** with a very long incubation period, Creutzfeldt–Jakob disease is presumably caused by a **pro**teinaceous **in**fectious particle, or **prion**, and is transmitted via corneal transplants, **dura mater allografts,** contaminated cadaveric growth hormone, or neurosurgical contamination. Lithium overdose may mimic signs and symptoms. The prion is resistant to normal modes of sterilization such as heat inactivation. It appears that the infectious particle uses itself to generate mutant conformations of endogenous protein. The protein is then immunogenic, causing destruction of neurons.

Treatment

Supportive therapy; usually fatal.

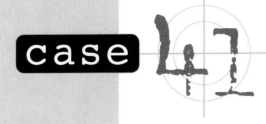

case 41

ID/CC	A 35-year-old woman known to have rheumatic mitral stenosis awakens in the morning to find the **right side of her body paralyzed.**
HPI	The patient also complains of **palpitations.** She has no history of fever, neck stiffness, vomiting, headache, or transient ischemic attacks (TIAs).
PE	VS: no fever; irregularly irregular pulse. PE: dense **right-sided hemiplegia; brisk reflexes on right side; right-sided Babinski** (EXTENSOR PLANTAR RESPONSE) **present;** fundus normal; loud S1; apical mid-diastolic murmur and opening snap.
Labs	ECG: presence of atrial fibrillation confirmed in addition to P-mitrale. Blood culture sterile; routine lab tests normal; clotting time, bleeding time, and PT normal.
Imaging	Echo: left atrial thrombus. CT: scan performed after 24 hours reveals **infarct in posterior limb of left internal capsule.**
Gross Pathology	Remote infarct with resorption of necrotic brain tissue leads to cyst formation.

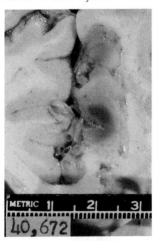

Figure 41-1. Remote cerebral infarction.

NEUROLOGY

81

case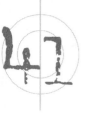

CVA, Capsular Infarct

Differential | Migraine
Focal seizure
Tumor
Conversion disorder

Discussion | Patients with mitral stenosis are prone to stasis, which can lead to the development of a thrombus in the heart. If the thrombus becomes instable, it can break away, causing thromboembolic phenomena. This includes the risk for ischemic bowel disease, as well as in this case a nonhemorrhagic stroke.

Treatment | Consider thrombolytic therapy if within 3 hours of symptoms and there is no evidence of hemorrhage. Patient then treated with heparin and eventually started on warfarin; therapy guided with PT. Management of atrial fibrillation with rate control agents such as beta-blockers; valvuloplasty or valve replacement after resolution of left atrial thrombus.

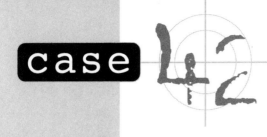

ID/CC	A **65-year-old** white **man** develops **sudden severe headache** and **left-sided hemiplegia**.
HPI	The patient is a **known hypertensive** and takes his medication irregularly; he now has both **urinary and fecal incontinence**.
PE	VS: **severe hypertension** (BP 210/180); no fever. PE: dense right-sided **hemiplegia**; funduscopic exam reveals presence of **papilledema** in addition to **hypertensive retinopathy**; right-sided **Babinski**; eyes deviated toward left; no meningeal signs present.
Labs	Routine labs normal; LP not done, since intracranial pressure (ICP) raised.
Imaging	CT, head: **focal hemorrhage** in right putamen region of basal ganglia, with blood demonstrated in the ventricles.

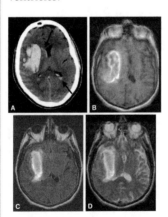

Figure 42-1. CT scan of a large basal ganglia hemorrhage.

Gross Pathology	Autopsy: mass of blood dissecting through parenchyma into deep structures of brain and ventricles.
Micro Pathology	Hypertensive changes seen in addition to putamenal hemorrhage; hyaline arteriolosclerosis; lipohyalinosis; Charcot–Bouchard aneurysms.

NEUROLOGY

case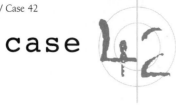

CVA, Hypertensive

Differential

Ruptured aneurysm
Focal seizure
Intracranial tumor
Spinal cord tumor

Discussion

Bleeding is most often caused by hypertension. In the presence of moderate to severe hypertension, **small penetrating arterioles** may rupture deep within the brain, causing a **hematoma** that displaces brain structures. Common sites are the **putamen, thalamus, pons,** and **cerebellum.**

Treatment

Supportive management to **reduce ICP** with ventilation control and osmotic diuretics, such as mannitol, and **blood pressure.** However, blood pressure should not be rapidly corrected.

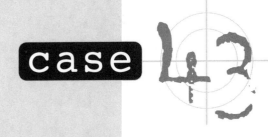

case 43

ID/CC   A 19-year-old woman, an Olympic horseback rider, is brought into the ER with **headache, confusion, weakness of the left side of her body, blurred vision, and projectile vomiting.**

HPI   Three hours ago, she hit the right side of her head when she fell from a horse during a training exercise. She **lost consciousness** for 1 minute and then appeared to have **recovered completely** before presenting with the symptomatology (LUCID INTERVAL).

PE   VS: BP mildly elevated; **bradycardia**. PE: **papilledema; right-sided mydriasis;** efferent pupillary reflex abnormality on right side; **deviation of right eyeball outward and downward** (RIGHT CN III PALSY); left-sided weakness; brisk reflexes on left side; **extensor plantar response** on left side.

Imaging   CT/MR, head: right temporal bone fracture; right-sided **lens-shaped** (convex) **hyperdense extra-axial fluid collection.**

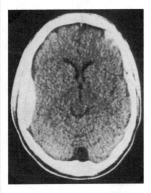

Figure 43-1. Convex extra-axial fluid collection.

Gross Pathology   Collection of blood between dura mater and skull with mass effect.

case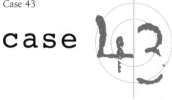

Epidural Hematoma

Differential

Alcoholism

Head injury

Cerebral abscess

Intracranial hemorrhage

Anisocoria

Discussion

The results of arterial bleeding (rupture of **middle meningeal artery**) are usually associated with skull fracture. Classically, the patient loses consciousness immediately after head injury but regains consciousness and remains asymptomatic for a variable period of time before symptoms worsen.

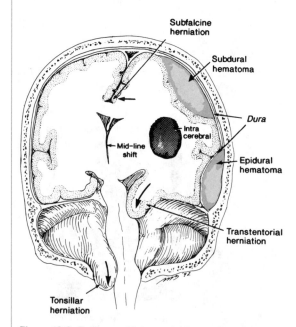

Figure 43-2. Patterns of intracranial hemorrhage and herniation.

Treatment

Emergent surgical evacuation.

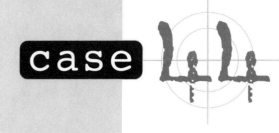

case

ID/CC A 19-year-old man visits his orthopedist because of a **wide-based gait** (ATAXIC GAIT), congenital **clubfoot,** and **abnormal lateral curvature of the spine** (SCOLIOSIS).

HPI For the past several years, he has had **increasing difficulty walking;** the process began subtly, but he is now incapable of participating in sports.

PE VS: tachycardia. PE: scoliosis of thoracic spine; pes cavus deformity of right foot; loss of vibration and joint position sense in hands and feet; areflexia in lower extremities; extensor plantar response (BABINSKI SIGN); ataxic gait; forceful "double" apical cardiac impulse; systolic ejection murmur; S4.

Labs ECG: left ventricular hypertrophy; inverted T waves. PCR reveals homozygosity for GAA repeat sequence.

Imaging Echo: evidence of hypertrophic obstructive cardiomyopathy.

Micro Pathology Marked loss of cells in posterior root ganglia and degeneration of peripheral sensory fibers; posterior and lateral columns of CNS also affected.

NEUROLOGY

case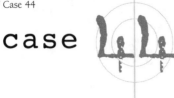

Friedreich Ataxia

Differential | Refsum disease
Abetalipoproteinemia
Spinocerebellar ataxia
Ataxia telangiectasia
Neurosarcoidosis

Discussion | The most common hereditary ataxia, Friedreich ataxia is an **autosomal recessive** disorder due to a defective gene on chromosome 9. It is due to trinucleotide repeat expansion in the frataxin gene.

■ TABLE 44-1 REPRESENTATIVE DISEASES ASSOCIATED WITH TRINUCLEOTIDE REPEATS

Disease	Location	Sequence	Normal Length	Premutation	Full Mutation
Huntington disease	4p16.3	CAG	10–35	—	40–100
Kennedy disease	Xq21	CAG	15–25	—	40–55
Spinocerebellar ataxia	6p23	CAG	20–35	—	45–80
Fragile X syndrome	Xq27.3	CGG	5–55	50–200	200–>1000
Myotonic dystrophy	19q13	CTG	5–35	37–50	50–4000
Friedreich ataxia	9q13	GAA	7–30	—	120–1700

Treatment | No specific treatment available.

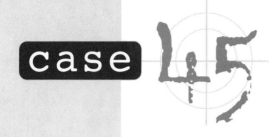

ID/CC	A 60-year-old white man complains of **headache** that is **worse in the morning** along with occasional **nausea and vomiting** for 6 weeks.
HPI	One day prior to presentation, he had an isolated **grand mal seizure**.
PE	Bilateral papilledema; loss of recent memory; **brisk deep tendon reflexes** on right side; **Babinski** on right side.
Imaging	CT/MR: **irregular enhancing left-sided mass** with **necrotic center; mass effect** and **surrounding edema**.
Gross Pathology	Hemorrhagic and necrotic tumor mass infiltrating left parietal lobe.

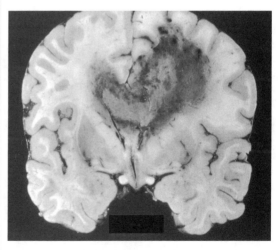

Figure 45-1. Irregularly colored mass with hemorrhage, cysts and necrosis, infiltrating both cerebral hemispheres.

Micro Pathology	Biopsy reveals presence of anaplastic cells with pleomorphism and endothelial proliferation; **foci of necrosis** surrounded by palisading.

89

case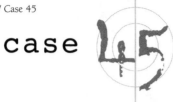

Glioblastoma Multiforme

Differential

Anaplastic astrocytoma
Cavernous malformation
Cerebral abscess
Oligodendroglioma
Intracranial hemorrhage
Intracranial metastasis

Discussion

Astrocytomas are graded according to differentiation; the **highest grade** (grade IV) **is glioblastoma multiforme.** It carries a poor prognosis.

Treatment

Surgical resection; chemotherapy; radiotherapy.

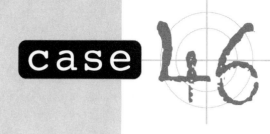

case 46

ID/CC   A 38-year-old man visits his family doctor complaining of **symmetric muscle weakness** that started **distally in his legs and ascended gradually,** now involving the trunk and arms.

HPI   A week ago he suffered from **diarrhea and fever** and was diagnosed with and treated for *Campylobacter* **enteritis.**

PE   **Symmetrical** proximal muscle **weakness** and **flaccidity** in lower limbs; absent deep tendon reflexes; normal sensory exam; normal cranial nerves.

Labs   Elevated gamma globulin. LP: **increased CSF protein concentration without cellular increase;** normal glucose. Nonreactive VDRL; **decreased nerve conduction velocity** indicative of **demyelination** on electrophysiologic studies.

Micro Pathology   Biopsy reveals presence of peripheral neurons with mononuclear (lymphocytic) infiltrate and demylination.

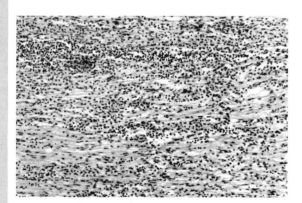

Figure 46-1. Diffuse mononuclear infiltrate around peripheral nerves.

case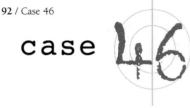

Guillain–Barré Syndrome

Differential | Inflammatory demyelinating polyradiculoneuropathy
Cauda equina syndrome
Conus medullaris syndrome
HIV neuropathy
Lyme disease
Myasthenia gravis
Organophosphate poisoning

Discussion | Guillain–Barré syndrome is a common cause of **polyneuropathy** in adults that is usually **preceded by** GI or respiratory **infection** or by specific illnesses such as Epstein–Barr, *Campylobacter* enteritis, and cytomegalovirus infection. **Respiratory paralysis** may occur, necessitating **mechanical ventilation.**

Treatment | Plasmapheresis; intensive care and respiratory support.

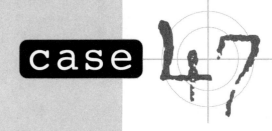

case 47

ID/CC	A 50-year-old man presents to the ER with **wild, flinging movements of his left arm and leg.**
HPI	He has been diagnosed with **diabetes and hypertension** but has taken his medications only irregularly. He is also a **chronic smoker.**
PE	Uncontrolled, violent, rapid flinging movements of left arm and leg; remainder of neurologic exam normal.
Labs	Lab tests reveal elevated blood glucose.
Imaging	CT (done at 48 hours): infarct in right **subthalamic nucleus.**

case 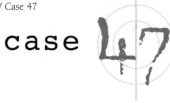 47

Hemiballismus

Differential

Acute hemichorea

Focal seizure

Tuberculous meningitis

Wilson disease

Discussion

Hemiballismus is characterized by forceful, flinging, and violent movements, primarily of the proximal parts of the limbs of one side of the body, which disappear during sleep. The most common etiology is that of a vascular event in the contralateral subthalamic nucleus; other causes include an expanding arteriovenous malformation, trauma, tumor, and multiple sclerosis. Most cases resolve spontaneously within 6 to 8 weeks; however, surgery may be indicated in cases of intractable involuntary movements.

■ TABLE 47-1 SYNDROMES ASSOCIATED WITH CEREBRAL INFARCTION

Artery occluded	Syndrome
Common carotid	Asymptomatic
Internal carotid	Ipsilateral blindness
	Contralateral hemiparesis and hemianesthesia
	Hemianopia
	Aphasia or denial and hemineglect
Middle cerebral	
Main trunk	Hemiplegia
	Hemianesthesia
	Hemianopia
	Aphasia or denial and hemineglect
Upper division	Hemiparesis and sensory loss (arm and face more affected than leg)
	Broca aphasia or denial and hemineglect
Lower division	Wernicke aphasia or nondominant behavior disorder without hemiparesis
Penetrating artery	Pure motor hemiparesis
Anterior cerebral	Hemiparesis and sensory loss affect leg more than arm
	Impaired responsiveness ("abulia" or "akinetic mutism"), especially if bilateral infarction
	Left-sided ideomotor apraxia or tactile anomia
Posterior cerebral	Cortical, unilateral; isolated hemianopia (or quadrantic field cut); alexia or color anomia
	Cortical, bilateral; cerebral blindness, with or without macular sparing
	Thalamic: pure sensory stroke; may leave anesthesia dolorosa with "spontaneous pain"
	Subthalamic nucleus: hemiballism
	Bilateral inferior temporal lobe: amnesia
	Midbrain: oculomotor palsy and other eye-movement abnormalities

Treatment

Phenothiazines and dopamine antagonists such as sulpiride and tetrabenazine may be of help.

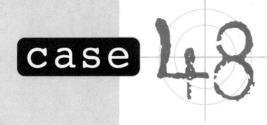

case 48

ID/CC	A **42-year-old** man presents with **depression,** poor memory, and **jerking movements** of the limbs and fingers.
HPI	His **father died of a similar** condition in which the symptoms progressively worsened, proceeding to dementia until his death at the age of 50.
PE	**Chorea;** psychiatric evaluation reveals **cognitive impairment** (inattention and poor concentration without memory loss) and depression; no other focal neurologic deficit found.
Imaging	MR, brain: degeneration of putamen and **caudate nucleus.** CT, brain: cerebral atrophy.
Gross Pathology	Loss of brain mass with striking **atrophy of caudate nucleus** and, less strikingly, putamen; secondary loss of neurons in globus pallidus; cortical atrophy most commonly occurs in frontal lobe.

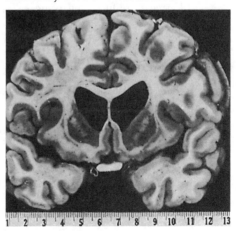

Figure 48-1. Atrophy of the caudate nuclei (arrow) with "bat wing" lateral ventricles.

Micro Pathology	Degeneration of spiny GABAergic neurons in the striatum leads to a net loss of inhibitory signals from the striatum.

NEUROLOGY

95

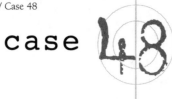

case

Huntington Chorea

Differential

Chorea gravidarum
Multiple sclerosis
Sydenham chorea
Paroxysmal dyskinesia
Hemiballismus

Discussion

Huntington chorea is an **autosomal dominant** disease whose gene locus is on chromosome 4. It is caused by expansion of a **trinucleotide repeat** (CAG) within the Huntington gene; expansion of the trinucleotide repeat leads to greater frequency of disease in successive generations (GENETIC ANTICIPATION). The onset of the disease is typically between 30 and 50 years of age, progressing to death within 15 to 20 years.

Treatment

No specific treatment available; supportive and symptomatic treatment; genetic counseling with regard to future offspring.

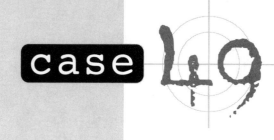

case 49

ID/CC	A 25-year-old man is brought to a neurologist with complaints of **inability to see on one side.**
HPI	Two months ago he suffered **right eye optic neuritis,** but his vision has significantly improved since then, although it is not completely normal.
PE	On lateral gaze in either direction, one eye does not adduct and the other has **nystagmus;** funduscopy reveals temporal pallor of right disk (due to atrophy of papillomacular fibers); visual field testing reveals right paracentral scotoma; **flexion of neck produces an electrical sensation that runs down back and into legs** (LHERMITTE SIGN).
Labs	LP: specific increase in CSF IgG concentration. Agarose electrophoresis reveals oligoclonal bands in IgG region of CSF. Evoked-potential studies of visual, auditory, and somatosensory pathways indicate impaired responses.
Imaging	MR, brain (T2W): investigation of choice; reveals **multiple, discrete, white-matter plaques.**
Gross Pathology	Sharply defined areas of gray discoloration (PLAQUES) of white matter that occur particularly frequently around the ventricles and in the corpus callosum.
Micro Pathology	Active plaques show evidence of myelin breakdown, lipid-laden macrophages, loss of oligodendrocytes, and relative preservation of axons; lymphocytes and mononuclear cells prominent at edges of plaques.

NEUROLOGY

case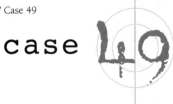

Internuclear Ophthalmoplegia

Differential

Multiple sclerosis

Brain stem infarction

Neurosyphilis

Lyme disease

Drug intoxication

Discussion

The following are suggestive of multiple sclerosis: (a) optic neuritis, whose early signs include diminished visual acuity, central or paracentral scotoma, hyperemia and edema of the optic disk, and a defective pupillary reaction to light; (b) internuclear ophthalmoplegia (due to demyelination of the medial longitudinal fasciculus); and (c) Lhermitte sign.

Treatment

Beta-interferon; immunosuppression (corticosteroids, azathioprine, cyclosporine), but success has been modest.

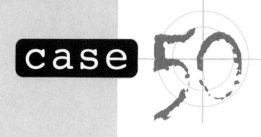

case **50**

ID/CC A 15-year-old boy is brought to a physician by his parents for an evaluation of recently observed **overindulgence in sexual activities.**

HPI The parents also report that the patient's behavior has recently changed markedly from **aggressive to extremely placid;** directed questioning reveals that he has now started **exploring things orally** and has developed a voracious appetite. He suffered from **herpes simplex encephalitis** a few months ago. There is no history of prior psychiatric illness in the patient or in the family.

PE Patient is in excellent health and is apparently unconcerned about his illness, displaying no reaction to parents' complaints; when physician attempts to shake his hand, patient begins to orally explore it; on seeing a nurse in doctor's room, he starts to masturbate.

Imaging MR/CT, head: **bilateral temporal lobe and amygdala damage.**

Gross Pathology Hemorrhagic necrotizing inflammation of the bilateral temporal lobes.

case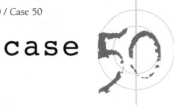

Klüver–Bucy Syndrome

Differential

Herpes encephalitis

Trauma

Cerebral vascular accident

Discussion

Klüver–Bucy syndrome is a syndrome of **hyperphagia, hypersexuality, placidity, and hyperorality.** In experimental animals, it results from **bilateral removal of the amygdala;** in humans, an incomplete picture is generally seen secondary to extensive temporal lobe damage, as may occur during herpes simplex encephalitis or in degenerative or posttraumatic brain damage.

Treatment

No specific treatment available.

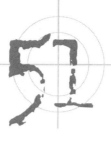

ID/CC A **6-year-old** boy is brought to the ER with acute-onset **projectile vomiting,** severe headache, and blurring of vision.

HPI The patient reports **unsteadiness of gait** that has progressively worsened over the past 2 months. He has no history of seizures, fever, or neck stiffness.

PE **Papilledema;** no meningeal signs; nystagmus in all directions of gaze; truncal ataxia; cranial nerves normal.

Labs CBC: mild anemia.

Imaging CT/MR, brain: homogeneous, enhancing **mass in cerebellar vermis** compressing and filling fourth ventricle; **dilated third and lateral ventricles.**

NEUROLOGY

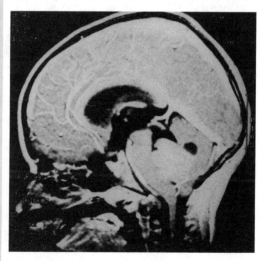

Figure 51-1. Large posterior fossa mass.

Gross Pathology Soft, well-circumscribed, light-grayish mass on cerebellar vermis.

Micro Pathology Once intracranial pressure (ICP) is controlled, CSF on lumbar puncture shows malignant cells; highly malignant tumor characterized by deeply staining nuclei with scant cytoplasm arranged in **pseudorosettes.**

101

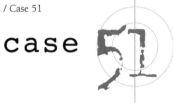

case

Medulloblastoma

Differential | Brain stem glioma
Craniopharyngioma
Hydrocephalus
Ependymoma
Low-grade astrocytoma

Discussion | A common tumor of **childhood** and the most prevalent brain tumor in children younger than 7 years of age, medulloblastoma is classified as a primitive neuroectodermal tumor (PNET).

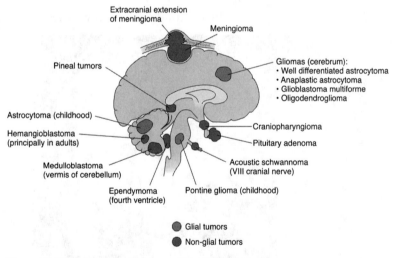

Figure 51-2. Distribution of common intracranial tumors.

Treatment | Entire neuraxis irradiation; surgical extirpation; chemotherapy.

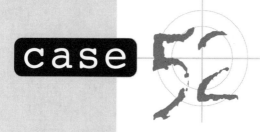

case 52

ID/CC A 40-year-old **man** complains that "the whole room seems to be spinning" (VERTIGO) while also experiencing ringing in the ears (TINNITUS) and nausea.

HPI The patient also complains of a **sense of fullness** in his ears and adds that his **hearing has progressively diminished** over the past few years. His symptoms were initially **unilateral but have now become bilateral.** His illness has run a course of **remissions and relapses.** He denies any weakness of the limbs and has no history of ear discharge or trauma.

PE VS: normal. PE: anxious; neurologic exam normal; caloric tests bilaterally normal.

Labs Pure-tone audiometry reveals **sensorineural hearing loss** that is more marked for **lower frequencies;** loudness recruitment present; short-increment sensitivity index (SISI) shows high score; VDRL negative.

Imaging MR/CT, head: normal (performed to rule out internal auditory canal pathology).

Micro Pathology **Gross distention of the endolymphatic system** (ENDOLYMPHATIC HYDROPS).

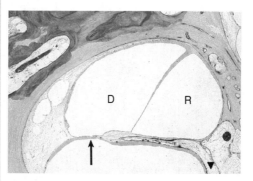

Figure 52-1. Marked distention of the cochlear duct (D). The Reissner membrane (R) is pushed back by endolymph hydrops. Neither the organ of corti (arrow) nor the spiral ganglion (arrowhead) is in its usual location.

case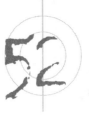

Ménière Disease

Differential

Migraine headache
Labyrinthitis
Otitis media
Salicylate toxicity
Low vestibular neuronitis

Discussion

Ménière disease is a disease of the inner ear characterized by **acute onset** and **recurrent attacks of vertigo**; it is often associated with nausea and vomiting **together with diminished hearing and tinnitus.** Although the exact etiology is unknown, endolymphatic hydrops (due to excess of endolymph in the scala media) has been linked to obstruction of resorption, defective membrane exchange, and increased endolymph inflow (secondary to allergy, vasomotor factors, or retained sodium and water).

Treatment

No specific treatment; symptomatic relief with **vestibular suppressants, diuretics,** and low-sodium diet. Surgical intervention is controversial.

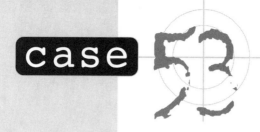

case 53

ID/CC	A 60-year-old **woman** is seen with complaints of difficulty walking and two episodes of **involuntary hand jerking** (PARTIAL SEIZURE).
HPI	Her attendant reveals that over the past few months her **memory has deteriorated**. She has slow mentation and **urinary incontinence**.
PE	Funduscopy reveals papilledema; deep tendon reflexes exaggerated; bilateral Babinski.
Labs	Routine laboratory tests normal.
Imaging	XR, skull: **hyperostosis** of left parietal bone and sagittal suture. CT (with contrast): left parietal **parasagittal tumor.** MR (gadolinium): **intense tumor enhancement; dural extension** and invasion into superior sagittal sinus.
Gross Pathology	Irregular, firm, **gritty mass arising superficially, indenting and compressing brain but not invading it.**

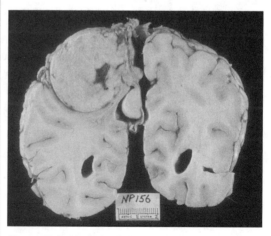

Figure 53-1. Mass that indents but does not infiltrate the brain parenchyma.

Micro Pathology	**Whorling pattern** of cells with regular, oval nuclei, indistinct cytoplasm, and **psammoma bodies.**

NEUROLOGY

105

case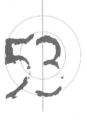

Meningioma

Differential	Complex partial seizure Craniopharyngioma Glioblastoma multiforme Neurofibromatosis Pituitary tumors
Discussion	Meningioma is a primary intracranial neoplasm arising from cells of the **arachnoid granulations**; it is characterized by **slow growth, benign behavior, and expansile rather than infiltrative growth.** Common sites involved include the cerebral convexity, parasagittal area (as in this case), sphenoid wing, olfactory groove, cerebellopontine angle, foramen magnum, and spinal cord. The tumor is usually solitary, is more common in women, and is found in middle and later ages. Multiple meningiomas may be found in patients with neurofibromatosis type 2.
Treatment	Surgical resection; radiation for unresectable cases.
Breakout Point	

Psammoma Bodies = Calcified Concretions Found in:
Meningiomas Papillary carcinoma of the thyroid Papillary serous cystadenocarcinoma of the ovaries

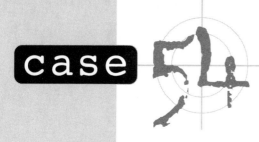

case 54

ID/CC A 59-year-old white woman presents with a **severe, dull retro-orbital headache,** vomiting, and **diplopia.**

HPI She has **smoked** two packs of cigarettes a day for 22 years and has been diagnosed with **lung cancer.**

PE VS: bradycardia; mild hypertension. PE: **papilledema** (due to increased intracranial pressure); **right pupillary reflex abnormality** in efferent pathway (due to right occulomotor nerve palsy).

Imaging CT/MR: round, discrete, **ring-enhancing lesion** in right frontal lobe; surrounding vasogenic edema; **shifting of midline structures to left** (>1-cm shift considered severe).

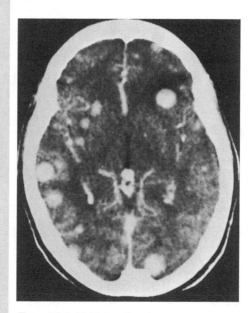

Figure 54-1. Multiple enhancing masses.

Micro Pathology Biopsy shows small cell carcinoma.

case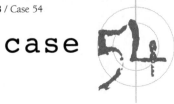

Metastatic Brain Tumor

Differential

Brain abscess
Hypertensive hemorrhage
CNS lymphoma
Meningioma
Toxoplasmosis

Discussion

Metastatic brain tumors are more common than primary brain tumors. Common primary cancers that result in intracranial metastasis are lung, breast, GI, and GU cancer and melanoma.

Treatment

Consider surgical resection; radiation therapy or radiosurgery; dexamethasone (to control intracranial pressure).

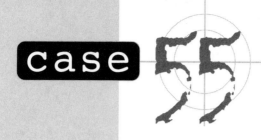

case 55

ID/CC A **20-year-old woman** complains of **recurrent, throbbing headaches** associated with profound **nausea and light sensitivity.**

HPI She has had similar headaches several times each year since the onset of her menstrual periods. The headaches occur on **one side of her head.** She also reports seeing "**flashing lights**" like lightning moving across her field of vision. **Stress, sleeplessness, and anxiety usually precipitate** these headaches. Her mother suffers from such headaches (positive family history).

PE VS: normal. PE: funduscopic exam and visual field testing normal; neurologic exam normal.

case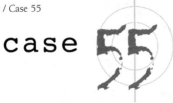

Migraine

Differential

Absence seizure
Cerebral aneurysm
Dissection syndromes
Tension headache
Meningitis
Pseudotumor cerebri

Discussion

Migraine headache is the **second most common** cause of **primary headache** (the most common in the United States is tension headache). In the United States, an estimated **17% of women** and 6% of men are affected by this disorder. The headache is characteristically preceded by a **prodrome** and is **episodic,** gradual in onset, **usually unilateral,** and most commonly in the **temporal area.** Precipitating factors may include menses, fasting, emotional stress, and foods containing tyramine, monosodium glutamate, or nitrites. The cause is unknown but appears to involve variations in cerebral blood flow and serotonergic pathways.

Treatment

Prophylactic therapy with avoidance of precipitating factors and drugs such as beta-blockers, tricyclic antidepressants, or calcium channel blockers; abortive therapy during acute attacks with NSAIDs, sumatriptan, ergotamine, or transnasal butorphanol.

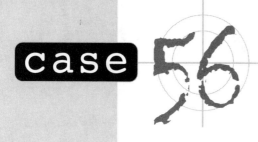

case 56

ID/CC A **36-year-old white** woman pays an emergency visit to her ophthalmologist because of **loss of central vision and pain on movement of her left eye** (due to optic neuritis); she also presents with scanning speech and **intention tremor** in the hands.

HPI She **emigrated** to the United States from **Sweden** 5 years ago. She has been suffering from **recurrent paresthesias in the hands, arms, and legs; weakness in the legs and arms; vertigo;** and **bladder urgency** (multiple unrelated neurologic symptoms).

PE Diminished visual acuity; central scotoma found on visual field charting; **hyperemia and edema** of left **optic disk;** defective afferent pupillary reaction to light in left eye (MARCUS GUNN PUPIL); **paresis of medial rectus muscle on lateral conjugate gaze but not on convergence** (BILATERAL INTERNUCLEAR OPHTHALMOPLEGIA); **nystagmus** in abducting eye; electrical sensation running down back and into legs produced by neck flexion (LHERMITTE SIGN); leg spasticity and increased deep tendon reflexes.

Labs LP: **marked increase in CSF IgG concentration;** presence of **oligoclonal bands** in IgG region on CSF agarose electrophoresis; CSF otherwise normal.

Imaging MR, brain: multiple discrete high T2 signal abnormalities in **periventricular** and other white matter areas (especially **corpus callosum**).

Gross Pathology Pathologic hallmark of disorder consists of distinctive small gray **plaques of demyelination** present in CNS white matter; optic neuritis.

Micro Pathology Demyelination and gliosis; lipid-laden macrophages.

case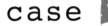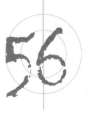

Multiple Sclerosis

Differential

Optic neuritis

Progressive multifocal leukoencephalitis

Chronic fatigue syndrome

Myasthenia gravis

Neurosarcoidosis

Spinocerebellar degeneration

Encephalitis

Discussion

Multiple sclerosis is an idiopathic demyelinating disorder whose course is marked by **intermittent remissions and exacerbations.**

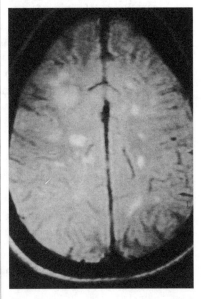

Figure 56-1. Multiple areas of demyelination seen on MRI.

Treatment

Symptomatic treatment; high-dose IV methylprednisone for acute optic neuritis; immunomodulators (β-interferon, glatiramer acetate) for reducing frequency of relapses; mitoxantrone for progressive disease.

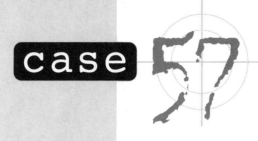

ID/CC A 25-year-old **woman** has had marked **weakness** and **drooping of the eyelids** (PTOSIS) in the evening for the past 4 weeks; she does not experience any weakness in the morning following a good night's sleep.

HPI She has also been suffering from **double vision** (DIPLOPIA) at the end of each day.

PE **Ptosis** develops on sustained elevation of eyelids; **dysphonia** develops as patient is asked to narrate complaints at length; **weakness of forward flexion of head develops after repetitive resistance to force;** patient could not maintain her upper limb in abducted position for more than a minute.

Labs **Clear-cut improvement in strength with edrophonium** administration. EMG: progressive decrement in voltage during repetitive, low-frequency stimulation of motor nerve. **Positive serum titer of antibodies to acetylcholine receptors.**

NEUROLOGY

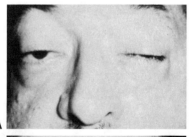

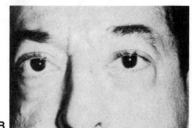

Figure 57-1. Characteristic ptosis (A) reversed by edrophonium injection (B).

case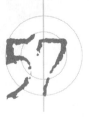

Myasthenia Gravis

Differential
Amyotrophic lateral sclerosis
Polymyositis
Lambert–Eaton myasthenic syndrome
Multiple sclerosis
Mitochondrial myopathies

Discussion
Myasthenia gravis is an **autoimmune disease** that is due to the development of specific **antibodies to one or more acetylcholine receptor subunits,** reducing the availability of acetylcholine receptors at the neuromuscular junction. **Thymoma** is present in 20% of cases.

Treatment
Acetylcholinesterase inhibitors (pyridostigmine); prednisone; thymectomy; plasmapheresis.

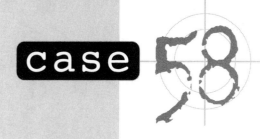

ID/CC   A 35-year-old man goes to a clinic because of **distal muscle weakness** in both upper and lower limbs and **gradual diminution of vision.**

HPI   His **father** suffered from a **similar muscular weakness.** The patient also suffers from mental retardation.

PE   **Frontal balding;** typical **facial wasting;** bilateral cataracts; **distal muscle weakness** in both upper and lower limbs; difficulty releasing grip after handshake; **percussion over tongue and thenar eminence reveals myotonia;** mildly reduced deep tendon reflexes; normal sensory exam; moderately **atrophic testicles;** equinovarus deformity of both feet.

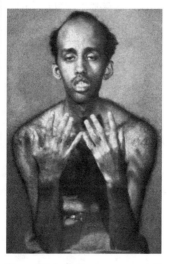

Figure 58-1. Patient on presentation.

Labs   **Decreased plasma IgG.** EMG: myopathic potentials.

Imaging   ECG: nonspecific ST-T changes.

Micro Pathology   Muscle biopsy reveals internal nuclei (nuclei in center of the fiber rather than in periphery), type I fiber atrophy, and ring fibers.

NEUROLOGY

115

case

Myotonic Dystrophy

Differential

Inclusion body myositis

Limb–girdle muscular dystrophy

Myotonia congenita

Parkinsonism

Cerebral palsy

Discussion

The most common form of muscular dystrophy among **whites**, myotonic dystrophy is transmitted as an **autosomal dominant** trait. It is associated with a genetic defect involving increased trinucleotide (AGC) repeats that encode for **myotonin protein kinase**; the myotonic dystrophy gene locus has been mapped at chromosome 19q13.3.

Treatment

Phenytoin; carbamazepine; quinidine; procainamide; acetazolamide; surgery required to correct foot deformities.

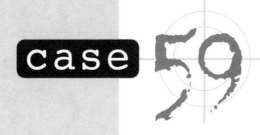

case 59

ID/CC	A **5-year-old boy** is referred to a specialist by his physician for evaluation of an **abdominal mass** and a recently noticed **left-sided orbital proptosis**.
HPI	His parents complain of weight loss, poor feeding, and a low-grade fever.
PE	PE: marked **cachexia**; left-sided orbital proptosis and ecchymoses; large, smooth **intra-abdominal mass palpable**.
Labs	Marked **elevation of urinary catecholamines** and metabolites vanillylmandelic acid (VMA) and homovanillic acid (HVA).
Imaging	CT, abdomen: **intra-abdominal mass arising from and obliterating left adrenal gland.** Nuc (bone scan): metastatic lytic lesion in left orbital region of skull.
Gross Pathology	Solid, round soft-tumor mass obliterating left adrenal gland; **gray on cut surface** showing extensive hemorrhage and necrosis with cyst formation.
Micro Pathology	Anaplastic, small, round-to-oval hyperchromatic cells with scant cytoplasm in sheets and at places forming **Homer–Wright pseudorosettes**; few ganglion cells seen; electron microscopy reveals presence of **neurosecretory granules**.

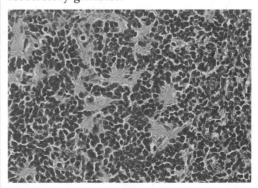

Figure 59-1. Homer–Wright pseudorosettes.

case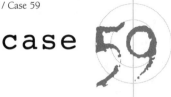

Neuroblastoma

Differential

Adrenal carcinoma

Adrenal hemorrhage

Pheochromocytoma

Wilms tumor

Rhabdomyosarcoma

Discussion

Neuroblastoma is a primary malignant neoplasm that arises from immature cells of the adrenal medulla and secretes catecholamines; it usually occurs in children under the age of 5 and presents with an abdominal mass. It is one of the small round blue cell tumors. Neuroblastomas most commonly originate in the adrenal glands but may also arise in the retroperitoneal sympathetic ganglia, pelvis, neck, or posterior mediastinum. Hutchinson neuroblastoma presents with extensive skull and orbital metastases that produce exophthalmos; metastases to lymph nodes, liver, lung, and bone are common.

Breakout Point

Small Round Blue Cell Tumors
(LEARRNNM) = lymphoma, Ewing sarcoma, ALL, retinoblastoma, rhabdomyosarcoma, neuroepithelioma, neuroblastoma, medulloblastoma

Treatment

Surgical resection; chemotherapy with cyclophosphamide and adriamycin.

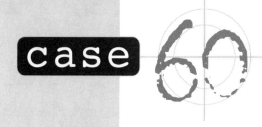

case 60

ID/CC	A 60-year-old man is seen by a neurologist for an evaluation of **deteriorating cognitive skills.**
HPI	Over the past few weeks, the patient has stayed in bed and has had urinary and bowel incontinence.
PE	Cognition impaired; impaired ambulation without evidence of primary motor, sensory, or cerebellar dysfunction (GAIT APRAXIA); deep tendon reflexes intact; pupils equal, round, and reactive to light and accommodation; plantars bilaterally flexor; fundus does not reveal any papilledema.
Labs	LP: normal opening pressure. Lab parameters within normal limits.
Imaging	CT: **ventricular enlargement with relatively little cortical atrophy.** Nuc, cisternography: persistent activity of radionuclide in lateral ventricles after 48 hours.

NEUROLOGY

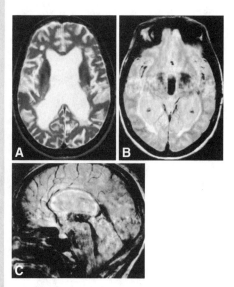

Figure 60-1. T2 weighted MRI with dilated lateral ventricles and no sulci effacement.

119

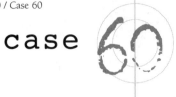

case 60

Normal Pressure Hydrocephalus

Differential

Alzheimer disease
Parkinson disease
Pick disease
Uremic encephalopathy
Multi-infarct dementia
Hallucinogen toxicity

Discussion

Pseudobulbar palsy is due to bilateral dysfunction of the corticobulbar tracts. In addition to dysphagia, dysarthria, and hyperactive gag reflexes, patients may experience episodes of spontaneous crying or laughter. In most patients, the cause of normal pressure hydrocephalus is not known, although it may follow a subarachnoid hemorrhage or meningitis (sometimes years later). The value of its early diagnosis lies in the fact that it is a **treatable dementia.**

Treatment

Insertion of a ventriculoperitoneal shunt.

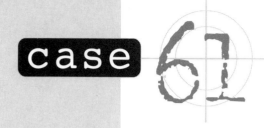
ID/CC	A 46-year-old white man complains to his internist of increasingly severe **headaches upon awakening** of a few months' duration; the headaches persist throughout the afternoon and are mild in the evenings.
HPI	While in the doctor's office, the patient suffers a **seizure** and is brought to the ER.
PE	Funduscopy reveals papilledema.
Labs	Normal.
Imaging	CT/MR: large **frontal lobe mass** with focal **nodular calcifications** with a **fried egg appearance**.

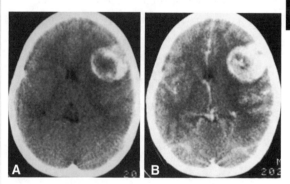

Figure 61-1. Mass with amorphous areas of calcification.

Gross Pathology	Calcified cystic tumor with gelatinous consistency and areas of necrosis and hemorrhage.
Micro Pathology	Tumor has **few anaplastic features**; regular cells aligned smoothly; spherical nuclei with finely granular chromatin, calcifications, and increased vascularity with areas of intratumoral bleeding.

NEUROLOGY

121

case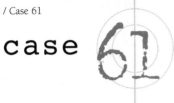

Oligodendroglioma

Differential

Malignant astrocytoma
Glioblastoma multiforme
Arteriovenous malformation
Meningioma
Brain abscess

Discussion

Usually low grade but occasionally anaplastic, oligo-dendrogliomas resemble astrocytomas in most respects but grow more slowly and are **more sensitive to chemotherapy**; calcification is noted in 90% of cases.

Treatment

Surgical resection/chemotherapy with radiation.

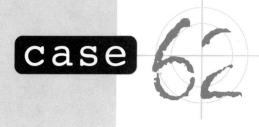
ID/CC   A 40-year-old man with a history of **insulin-dependent diabetes mellitus** (IDDM) presents with **tingling, numbness, burning, and aching in the lower legs and feet.**

HPI   The discomfort is particularly prominent at night and is often **relieved by walking.** A hoop over the feet to prevent contact with bedclothes is often helpful. The patient takes **insulin** irregularly.

PE   Mild weakness; mild **distal sensory loss** and **loss of position and vibration sense** in both legs; bilaterally reduced ankle and knee jerks. Patient has a large ulcerated lesion on the foot.

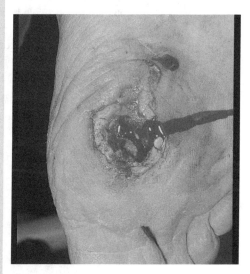

Figure 62-1. Well-demarcated, hemorrhagic ulcer on the sole, with exposed subcutaneous fat.

Labs   Nerve conduction velocities slowed. EMG: features of **denervation.** Elevated glycosylated hemoglobin levels indicate poor blood sugar control.

NEUROLOGY

case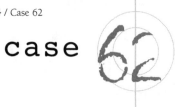

Peripheral Neuropathy—Diabetic

Differential

Alcoholic neuropathy
Nutritional neuropathy
Vasculitis
Thyroid disease
Amyloid neuropathy
Vitamin B$_{12}$ deficiency

Discussion

The neuropathy experienced by patients with long-term diabetes is one of the most distressful components of the disease. At first, it starts as pain and abnormal sensations in the extremities. Fine touch and proprioception are eventually lost. As such, normal noxious stimuli provided by minor traumas go unnoticed. Patients develop painless destructive lesions of the feet and joints. Ultimately, these lead to portals for systemic infection. Amputations of involved extremities are common.

Treatment

Tricyclic antidepressants, carbamazepine, and gabapentin may be effective for symptom control; strict glycemic control to slow progression. Amputation as necessary.

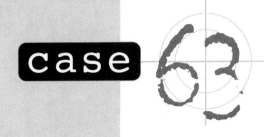

case 63

ID/CC A 35-year-old man who has been diagnosed with **multiple sclerosis** visits his physician with complaints of **difficulty swallowing** (DYSPHAGIA) and **nasal regurgitation** of food.

HPI Six months ago he suffered an attack of retrobulbar neuritis; 2 months ago he developed **spastic weakness of both lower limbs.**

PE Speech is monotonous, slurred, and high-pitched ("DONALD DUCK" DYSARTHRIA); he dribbles from mouth; cannot protrude his **tongue, which lies on the floor of the mouth and is small and spastic;** palatal movements absent; jaw jerk exaggerated; patient is emotionally labile.

Imaging MR, brain: multiple focal white-matter plaques.

case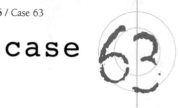

Pseudobulbar Palsy

Differential

Huntington disease
Stroke
Amyotrophic lateral sclerosis
Multiple sclerosis
Brain tumor

Discussion

The common causes of pseudobulbar palsy include bilateral cerebrovascular accidents involving the **internal capsule,** motor neuron disease, and multiple sclerosis.

Treatment

General management of multiple sclerosis; no specific treatment available.

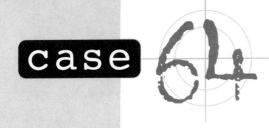

case 64

ID/CC	A 40-year-old man **dies** shortly after being brought to the emergency room with the "**most severe headache of his life.**"
HPI	His father died of chronic renal failure at the age of 45.
PE	Papilledema; nuchal rigidity.
Imaging	CT, head: **hyperdense blood** in cisterns and sulci.
Gross Pathology	Brain reveals staining of inferior surfaces of brainstem, cerebellum, and cerebral hemispheres with fresh blood due to congenital berry aneurysm rupture; both kidneys reveal polycystic changes; multiple cysts seen in liver.

NEUROLOGY

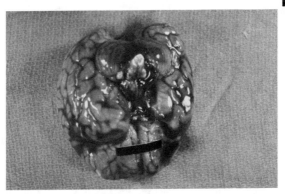

Figure 64-1. Diffuse blood staining the inferior surfaces of the brainstem, cerebellum, and cerebral hemispheres.

case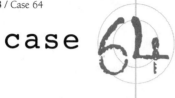

Subarachnoid Hemorrhage

Differential
Encephalitis
Cluster headache
Migraine headache
Hypertensive emergency
Temporal arteritis
Hemorrhagic stroke

Discussion
In this case, hemorrhage was caused by a ruptured intracranial aneurysm in a patient with **autosomal dominant polycystic kidney disease.** Other causes of subarachnoid hemorrhage include AV malformation and trauma.

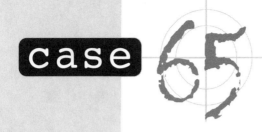

ID/CC A 30-year-old black man complains of **constant bifrontal headache** and **blurred vision** of 3-week duration.

HPI He has had mild intermittent **frontal headaches for the past 8 months** and has become **irritable**; for the past month he has been **extremely drowsy** and often sleeps for 30 hours at a time. Ten months ago, **he fell from a moving vehicle** and **lacerated his scalp**.

PE **Bilateral papilledema; dilated left pupil**; right spastic hemiparesis; deep tendon reflexes on right side are brisk; **right-sided Babinski**; no meningeal signs present.

Labs LP contraindicated due to raised intracranial pressure.

Imaging CT, head: **hyperdense crescentic extra-axial fluid collections (early); hypodense fluid collection with thick membranes (late).**

Gross Pathology Old blood encased in thick adherent brown membranes.

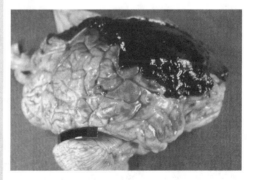

Figure 65-1. Large, well-demarcated accumulation of clotted blood beneath the dura, confined by the dural attachments.

Micro Pathology Outer membrane composed of granulation and fibrous tissue with hemosiderin; inner membrane shows fibrous tissue only.

129

case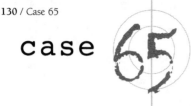

Subdural Hematoma

Differential

Epidural hematoma
Meningitis
Subdural empyema
Intracranial neoplasm
Ischemic stroke

Discussion

Subdural hematoma is a traumatic lesion character-ized by accumulation of blood between the dura and arachnoid. It is caused by **laceration of the bridging veins** and results in **displacement of the brain** and possible **cerebral herniations.**

Treatment

Surgical drainage of hematoma.

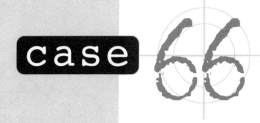

case **66**

ID/CC	A 30-year-old man is referred to a neurologist because of progressive **anesthesia and weakness of both arms, occipital headaches,** and a **stiff gait.**
HPI	He has no history of significant trauma in the past.
PE	Bilateral motor weakness of the hands and forearm; **lack of pain and temperature sensation in both hands and arms** (due to spinothalamic tract involvement) **but preserved position and tactile sensation** (dorsal columns uninvolved and proprioceptive sensation spared); unimpaired pain and temperature sensation below arms; **thenar muscles** of both hands **atrophied; areflexia in both upper limbs;** brisk deep tendon reflexes in both lower limbs.
Labs	Normal.
Imaging	MR/CT, spine: **cystic dilatation within central cervical cord.**

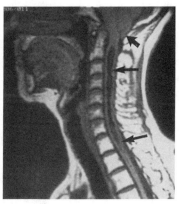

Figure 66-1. Central cord cavitation seen between long arrows on MRI.

Gross Pathology	Spinal cord shows **central cavitation** in longitudinal and cleftlike fashion.
Micro Pathology	Hydromyelia is lined by ependymal tissue; syringomyelia is not.

NEUROLOGY

case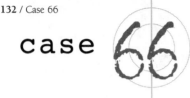

Syringomyelia

Differential | Amyotrophic lateral sclerosis
Cervical spondylosis
Ependymoma
Spinal cord infarction
Epidural abscess
Multiple sclerosis

Discussion | Syringomyelia may be primary (associated with **Arnold–Chiari malformation**) or acquired (post-traumatic, postinflammatory, tumor-associated).

Treatment | Surgery and neurorehabilitation.

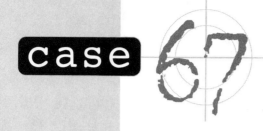
ID/CC A **79-year-old** white woman complains of a **throbbing, unilateral headache** that is most severe around her forehead and temples.

HPI She has had recurrent bouts of **fever** over the past year and also complains of **malaise** and **muscle aches**. She reports some weight loss and occasional **vision problems** in her right eye. She also reports **jaw pain when she is eating** (JAW CLAUDICATION).

PE VS: fever. PE: **nodular enlargement of temporal artery with tenderness.**

Labs CBC: normal WBC count; mild anemia. **Markedly elevated ESR**, usually >50 mm/hour.

Gross Pathology Swollen, cordlike, segmentally nodular temporal artery.

Micro Pathology **Granulomatous** inflammatory infiltrate of media and adventitia on **temporal artery biopsy**; fragmentation of internal elastic lamina with multinucleated giant cells and fibrotic patches.

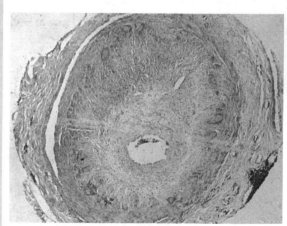

Figure 67-1. Granulomatous inflammation of the media with numerous multinucleated giant cells along degenerated internal elastic lamina. Intimal fibrosis with luminal narrowing.

RHEUMATOLOGY

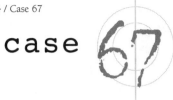

case 67

Temporal Arteritis

Differential
Glaucoma
Migraine headache
Retinal artery occlusion
Transient ischemic attack

Discussion
Temporal arteritis is the most **common vasculitis** in the United States; it frequently **coexists with polymyalgia rheumatica** and carries a risk of ipsilateral **blindness** due to thrombosis of the **ophthalmic artery**. Diagnosis and treatment are based on clinical grounds, because biopsy is positive in only 60% of cases.

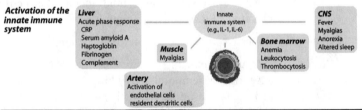

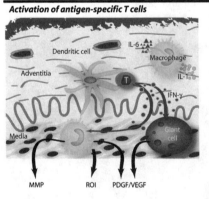

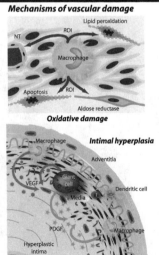

Figure 67-2. Pathogenesis of temporal arteritis.

Treatment
Steroids should be started empirically before biopsy confirmation to **prevent blindness**.

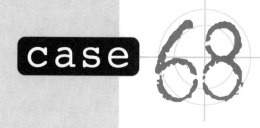

case 68

ID/CC	An 18-year-old man presents with **headache, ataxia, and progressive loss of vision.**
HPI	His **father** died of metastatic **bilateral renal cell carcinoma** at a relatively **young** age.
PE	**Cerebellar ataxia; nystagmus;** past-pointing and **inability to perform rapid alternating movements** (DYSDIADOCHOKINESIA); funduscopic exam reveals presence of **retinal hemangiomas** and moderate papilledema (due to increased intracranial pressure).
Labs	UA: normal (hematuria may signal renal cell carcinoma).
Imaging	CT/MR, head: **cerebellar solid/cystic lesion** with **enhancing mural nodule.** CT, abdomen: **renal, hepatic, and pancreatic cysts.**

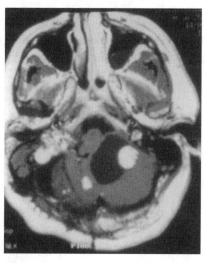

Figure 68-1. MRI demonstrating multiple enhancing cystic lesions.

Gross Pathology	**Hemangioblastomas** of cerebellum and retina; tumor occasionally located in medulla or cervical spinal cord.

135

case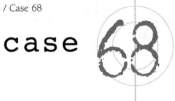

Von Hippel–Lindau Disease

Differential

Multiple endocrine neoplasia
Polycystic kidney disease
Tuberous sclerosis
Colloid cysts
Arachnoid cysts

Discussion

Von Hippel–Lindau disease is a rare **autosomal dominant** neurocutaneous dysplasia. The gene has been linked to the raf-1 oncogene on chromosome 3 and has a variable penetrance and delayed expression. The condition is **associated with renal cell carcinoma** that is often multifocal or bilateral.

Breakout Point

> Von Hippel–Lindau (VHL) **3** words = Chromosome **3**

Treatment

Surgical removal of tumor; photocoagulation for treatment of retinal lesions.

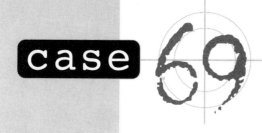

case 69

ID/CC	A **24-year-old man** visits his family doctor complaining of **low back pain and stiffness** of the spine for almost 1 year, increasing in severity.
HPI	The back stiffness is eased by a hot shower, and worsens after prolonged inactivity.
PE	**Stooped posture**; loss of lumbar lordosis and **fixed kyphosis; tenderness over sacroiliac joints**; reduced chest expansion; prominent abdomen.
Labs	Elevated ESR; **negative rheumatoid tests; positive HLA-B27.**
Imaging	XR, plain: sclerosis and blurring of margins of **sacroiliac joints; fusion of vertebrae** ("BAMBOO SPINE") in long-standing cases.

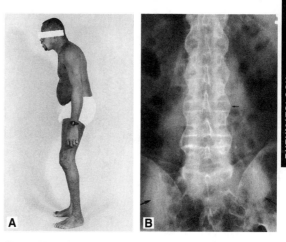

Figure 69-1. Posturing of patient (A) and bamboo spine (B).

Gross Pathology	Calcification of intervertebral disks and longitudinal ligaments.
Micro Pathology	Similar to rheumatoid arthritis, but in different location and no rheumatoid nodules.

RHEUMATOLOGY

case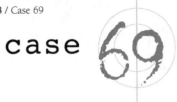

Ankylosing Spondylitis

Differential
Lumbar disk disease
Psoriatic arthritis
Reactive arthritis
Rheumatoid arthritis
Enteropathic arthropathies

Discussion
Also called Marie–Strümpell disease and associated with **HLA-B27**, this inflammatory arthritis with eventual ankylosis of the spine is typically seen in young men; long-standing cases may present with **iritis** and **aortic insufficiency.** Ankylosing spondylitis is also associated with Reiter syndrome and inflammatory bowel disease.

Treatment
Physical therapy; NSAIDs; sulfasalazine.

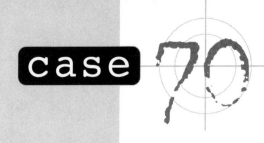

case 70

ID/CC A 55-year-old man is brought into the emergency department **diaphoretic** and **ashen** in appearance.

HPI He is an experienced pilot who was on a **cross-country flight** from New York to California. His ascent was uneventful to an altitude of **30,000 feet** above mean sea level in an unpressurized airplane. After 1 hour at this cruising altitude (and while on supplemental oxygen), the pilot noticed a gradual onset of **weakness and paresthesias of the right arm**. These symptoms progressively worsened to involve both arms.

PE VS: normal. PE: **disoriented and confused**; normal cardiac and pulmonary exam; neurologic exam revealed severe flexor weakness at the right elbow and wrist, numbness of the forearm, and impaired fine motor control.

Labs CBC/Lytes: normal. Ventilation-perfusion scan shows no V-Q mismatch. ABGs (at room air): normal.

Imaging CXR: mild increase in interstitial markings. Consider head CT scan if mental status changes do not improve with hyperbaric repressurization.

case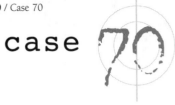

Decompression Sickness

Differential

Anaphylaxis
Pulmonary embolism
Hyperventilation syndrome
Myocardial infarction
Heat stroke

Discussion

Decompression sickness, also referred to as **Caisson disease,** occurs when a person is subjected to a rapid reduction in ambient pressure, resulting in the formation of dissolved bubbles of nitrogen within body tissues ("the bends"). DCS can result from high-altitude exposure (i.e., an unpressurized aircraft at >29,000 feet altitude) or from work in pressurized tunnels or caissons, and is **most commonly** associated with **compressed-air** (SCUBA) **diving.**

Treatment

Initial management with **hydration, 100% oxygen delivery by mask, and transfer to a hyperbaric chamber for compression therapy.** Serious cases of DCS may require intubation and pressor agents. **Compression therapy** is the definitive treatment, and treatment should be started as soon as possible.

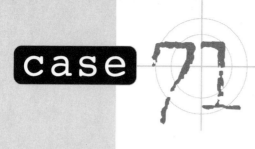
ID/CC   A 52-year-old white **woman** complains to her family doctor of **difficulty climbing** steps for the past 6 months and difficulty washing her hair for the past 2 weeks.

HPI   She states that she does not feel tired or short of breath but that her legs and arms "just will not cooperate." She also complains of intermittent fever.

PE   **Periorbital edema** with purplish discoloration (HELIOTROPE RASH); **butterfly rash** on face and neck; Raynaud phenomenon; **scaling of skin with redness around knuckles** (GOTTRON LESIONS); **proximal muscle weakness with tenderness** in all four extremities.

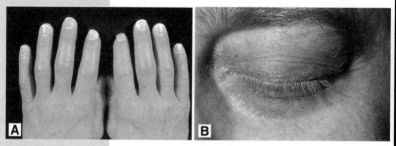

Figure 71-1. Gottron lesions (A) and heliotrope rash (B).

Labs   CBC: mild leukocytosis. **Elevated serum CK**; elevated aldolase; elevated ESR; **antinuclear antibodies (ANAs)**. EMG: spontaneous fibrillation.

Gross Pathology   Muscle edema progressing to muscle atrophy and fibrosis.

Micro Pathology   Muscle biopsy shows lymphocytic infiltration, primarily in a perivascular fashion but also between muscle fibers on muscle biopsy; atrophy and fibrosis seen.

RHEUMATOLOGY

case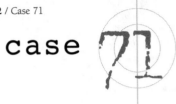

Dermatomyositis

Differential | Graft-versus-host disease
Hypothyroidism
Sarcoidosis
Lupus erythematosus
Psoriasis

Discussion | Dermatomyositis is an idiopathic disorder primarily affecting older females; it is frequently associated with malignancy (e.g., lung cancer). Patients have characteristic ANAs to antihistidyl transfer RNA [t-RNA] synthetase (Anti-Jo-1).

Treatment | Corticosteroids; methotrexate; azathioprine.

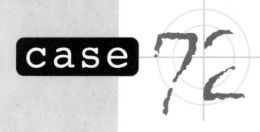

case 72

ID/CC	A 2-year-old boy presents with a persistent **low-grade fever, skin rash, and painful swelling of both knees.**
HPI	He has no history of sore throat, pedal edema/orthopnea, nocturnal dyspnea, or involuntary movements.
PE	VS: fever. PE: extensive erythematous maculopapular rash; generalized lymphadenopathy; hepatosplenomegaly; arthritis of both knees; no subcutaneous nodules; no evidence of carditis; no Roth spots on funduscopy.

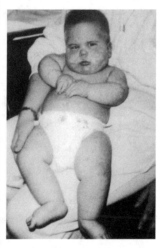

Figure 72-1. Florid erythematous maculopapular rash that appeared with fever.

Labs	CBC/PBS: leukocytosis; normocytic, normochromic anemia. Elevated ESR; blood cultures sterile; ASO titers normal; throat swab sterile; **rheumatoid factor negative;** leukocytosis with **elevated proteins and markedly low glucose and complement levels** on synovial fluid analysis. ECG: normal.
Imaging	XR, knees: effusion and soft tissue swelling. Echo: no vegetations or valvular disease.

case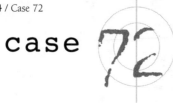

Juvenile Rheumatoid Arthritis

Differential

Acute lymphoblastic leukemia

Bacterial endocarditis

Kawasaki disease

Sarcoidosis

Systemic lupus erythematosus

Fifth disease

Discussion

Juvenile rheumatoid arthritis (JRA) most commonly affects the knee joint. Patients with JRA should undergo periodic ophthalmologic exams to carefully monitor for the onset of **iridocyclitis,** which can lead to blindness.

Treatment

NSAIDs; corticosteroids.

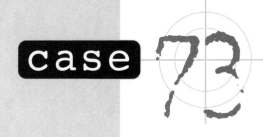
case 72

ID/CC   A 42-year-old woman presents with **dysphagia, butterfly rash**, arthralgias, myalgias, **skin stiffness,** swelling of the fingers, **proximal muscle weakness,** and **chronic pain in the finger joints.**

HPI   She has had these symptoms intermittently over the years, but they have worsened over the past year.

PE   VS: BP normal. PE: erythematous rash over face in butterfly distribution; **sclerodactyly;** telangiectasias in periungual areas; **nonerosive arthritis of wrist and ankle joints; proximal muscle weakness** and tenderness; weakness of neck muscles; no sensory loss; normal tendon reflexes; positive **Raynaud phenomenon.**

Labs   Elevated ESR; diffuse hypergammaglobulinemia; **positive rheumatoid factor;** high titer of antinuclear antibodies (speckled pattern); **strongly positive test for antibody to RNP antigen** (most typical finding); anti-Smith antibody negative; anti-dsDNA antibody negative; normal complement levels; elevated **serum CPK** levels; muscle biopsy and EMG suggestive of polymyositis; **normal RFTs.**

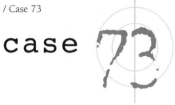

case

Mixed Connective Tissue Disease

Differential | Dermatomyositis
Polymyositis
Rheumatoid arthritis
Lupus erythematosus
Bacterial sepsis

Discussion | Mixed connective tissue disorder (MCTD) includes characteristics of **one or more traditional connective tissue diseases at the same time,** thus making it hard to label as one or the other. These disorders include systemic lupus erythematosus, scleroderma, rheumatoid arthritis, and polymyositis.

■ TABLE 73-1 ANTI-NUCLEAR ANTIBODIES AND DISEASE

ANA Pattern (FANA)	Usual Nuclear Antigens	Disease Correlation
Homogeneous (diffuse)	Histone	DILE
	Histone—DNA	SLE and other autoimmune diseases
Peripheral (rim)	dsDNA	SLE
Nucleolar	RNA	Scleroderma
		SLE
Speckled	Sm	SLE
	RNP	MCTD, SLE
	SS-A (Ro)	SS, SLE (classic, neonatal, SCLE)
	SS-B (La)	SLE, SS
	Centromere	CREST

ANA, antinuclear antibody; DILE, drug-induced lupus erythematosus; Sm, Smith antigen; RNP, ribonucleoprotein; dsDNA, double-stranded DNA; CREST, **c**alicinosis, **R**aynaud phenomenon, **e**sophageal dysmotility, **s**clerodactyly, **t**elangiectasia syndrome; FANA, fluorescent patterns of ANA; MCTD, mixed connective tissue disease; SCLE, subacute cutaneous LE; SLE, systemic lupus erythematosus; SS, Sjögren syndrome.

Treatment | Corticosteroids and NSAIDs.

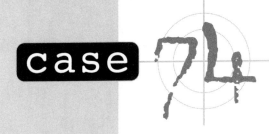

case 74

ID/CC	An **18-year-old man** presents with a **fracture of the shaft of the femur following a minor fall.**
HPI	He also complains of **facial asymmetry,** deviation of the angle of the mouth, drooling of saliva, and inability to whistle. **His father suffers from a bone disease.**
PE	Fracture of shaft of left femur; right facial nerve palsy, lower motor neuron type (entrapment neuropathy).
Labs	**Serum acid phosphatase and creatine kinase (brain isozyme) increased;** serum PTH increased; serum calcium and calcitriol normal. CBC: anemia.
Imaging	XR: **generalized symmetric osteosclerosis; "Erlenmeyer flask" deformity** of distal left femur in addition to fracture of shaft; alternating dense and lucent bands seen in metaphyses; cranium thickened and dense; paranasal and nasal sinuses underpneumatized; vertebrae show, on lateral view, **"bone in bone," "rugger-jersey"** appearance.
Micro Pathology	Histopathologic studies reveal profound **deficiency of osteoclast function** and **primary spongiosa** (calcified cartilage deposited during endochondral bone formation) occurring away from growth plate.

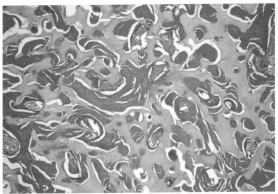

Figure 74-1. "Rugger-jersey" appearance of bone.

RHEUMATOLOGY

147

case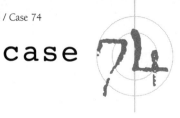

Osteopetrosis

Differential

Hypoparathyroidism
Pseudohypoparathyroidism
Lead toxicity
Paget disease
Myeloproliferative disease

Discussion

Also know as marble bone disease, osteopetrosis is a **defect in bone resorption** secondary to **impaired osteoclast action,** which is the key factor in the pathogenesis of osteopetrosis.

Treatment

Steroid therapy with low-calcium, high-phosphate diet; management of fracture and surgical decompression of facial nerve.

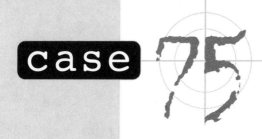

ID/CC A **60-year-old woman** visits her physician complaining of severe low back pain after a fall from her bed.

HPI Onset of **menopause** was at 48 years. The patient is **not receiving hormone replacement therapy;** she suffered a Colles fracture last year that is malunited. Directed history reveals **loss of height and a mild hunchback deformity.**

PE Patient thin; kyphosis noted; percussion over dorsolumbar spine exquisitely tender; right wrist shows malunited Colles fracture.

Labs Serum calcium, phosphates, alkaline phosphatase, and PTH within normal limits.

Imaging XR, dorsolumbar spine: loss of vertical height of L4 vertebra (due to collapse and compression fracture) and kyphosis. DEXA: T score $\gtrsim 2.5$.

Gross Pathology **Thin cortex; thin trabeculae, reduced in number,** resulting in increased medullary space; obvious fracture with healing and deformity; **collapse of vertebral bodies** with kyphoscoliosis.

Micro Pathology Bone biopsy: thin but normally formed cortex and trabeculae; normal calcification; trabeculae very slender; microfractures and fracture healing may be evident.

RHEUMATOLOGY

case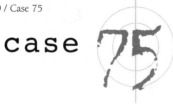

Osteoporosis

Differential | Hyperparathyroidism
Multiple myeloma
Renal osteodystrophy
Bone metastasis
Rickets

Discussion | Osteoporosis is characterized by a **reduction of total skeletal mass due to increased bone resorption** (bone formation is normal) with greater loss of trabecular than compact bone; it results in a predisposition to pathologic fracture. Common fracture sites are the thoracic and lumbar spine, distal forearm, and proximal femur.

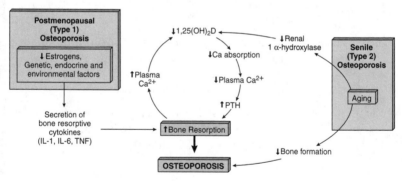

Figure 75-1. Pathogenesis of osteoporosis.

Treatment | **Calcium and vitamin D supplementation; estrogens** (shown to halt progressive bone loss); **bisphosphonates;** calcitonin; teriparatide; **exercise** (weight bearing acts as stimulus to bone formation); bracing of spine to prevent further fractures and deformity in a severely osteoporotic spine.

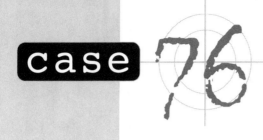
case 76

ID/CC	A 44-year-old man with a history of hypertension develops sudden abdominal pain (due to mesenteric thrombosis) far more severe than prior episodes.
HPI	The patient had a previous episode of hematuria with peripheral edema that was diagnosed as glomerulonephritis. He has a history of intermittent fever, malaise, myalgia, arthralgia, and other vague systemic symptoms.
PE	**Livedo reticularis;** subcutaneous nodules of forearms and finger pads; painful, tympanic abdomen; purpuric spots in lower legs; **radial and peroneal nerve involvement** (MONONEURITIS MULTIPLEX).
Labs	CBC: marked neutrophilic **leukocytosis** with eosinophilia. Elevated ESR; **presence of HBsAg; positive P-ANCA.**
Imaging	Angio, renal: **multiple small aneurysms** and **infarcts.**
Gross Pathology	Fibrinoid necrotizing inflammatory infiltrate of media and adventitia of small and medium-size vessels in segmental fashion, with thrombosis and possible aneurysm formation.
Micro Pathology	Segmental areas of **fibrinoid necrosis** with neutrophilic infiltration of arterial wall.

RHEUMATOLOGY

case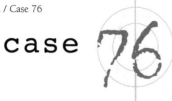

Polyarteritis Nodosa

Differential

Cholesterol embolism
Cryoglobulinemia
Infectious endocarditis
Lupus erythematosus
Dermatomyositis

Discussion

Polyarteritis nodosa is a **type III hypersensitivity reaction** characterized by **multisystem** involvement. **Renal involvement** is most common, but other presentations include pericarditis, myocardial infarction, retinal occlusion, and asthma.

Treatment

Steroids and other immunosuppressive agents.

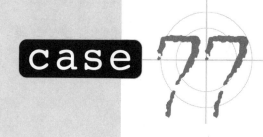
case 77

ID/CC A **70-year-old woman** is seen with complaints of **inability to comb her hair, put on her coat, and get up from her chair for the past 6 months.**

HPI She complains of **shoulder and pelvic area stiffness** and pain (especially during **morning hours**), fever, malaise, and fatigue.

PE VS: low-grade fever. PE: pallor; stiff, deliberate movements; affected joints show restricted movement; **muscle strength normal;** remainder of physical exam normal.

Labs CBC: **normochromic anemia. ESR markedly elevated;** other acute-phase reactants such as fibrinogen and β_2-globulin levels increased.

Imaging XR: normal.

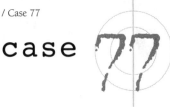

case

Polymyalgia Rheumatica

Differential

Amyloidosis
Fibromyalgia
Depression
Osteoarthritis
Polymyositis

Discussion

Polymyalgia rheumatica is characterized by **aching and morning stiffness** in the shoulder and hip girdles, the proximal extremities, the neck, and the torso; the spectrum of disease includes giant cell arteritis. Mean age at onset is 70; women are affected twice as often as men. A strong association with **HLA-DR4** has been observed. Some cases recur and some patients become steroid dependent. Approximately 15% of polymyalgia rheumatica patients develop giant cell arteritis (temporal arteritis).

Treatment

Low-dose oral steroids; watch for development of giant cell arteritis, which threatens vision in up to one-third of patients.

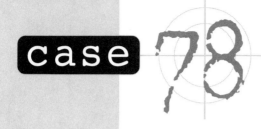

case 78

ID/CC   A 37-year-old white woman complains of **increasing weakness** for several months, especially when climbing stairs and combing her hair.

HPI   She also complains of **difficulty holding her neck upright.** For the past few weeks, she has also had **difficulty swallowing.**

PE   **Atrophy of neck, shoulder, and thigh muscles; motor weakness in all proximal muscle groups; no sensory deficit;** deep tendon reflexes reduced.

Labs   **Markedly elevated serum CPK levels; antinuclear antibodies (ANAs) demonstrable;** elevated serum transaminases and aldolase. EMG: markedly increased insertional activity; polyphasic low-amplitude motor unit action potentials with abnormally low recruitment.

Gross Pathology   Muscle edema progressing to muscle atrophy and fibrosis.

Micro Pathology   Biopsy from thigh muscles reveals **inflammatory infiltrate** in muscle, destruction of muscle fibers, and perivascular infiltrate of mononuclear cells; residual muscle fibers small.

RHEUMATOLOGY

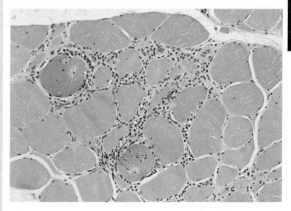

Figure 78-1. Mononuclear infiltrate into muscle bundles.

155

case 78

Polymyositis

Differential | Amyotrophic lateral sclerosis
Rheumatoid arthritis
Hypokalemia
Myasthenia gravis
Trichinosis

Discussion | Polymyositis is frequently seen as a **paraneoplastic** manifestation of ovarian, breast, uterine, or intestinal malignancy. An associated neoplasm should always be sought.

Treatment | High-dose glucocorticoids; methotrexate; azathioprine.

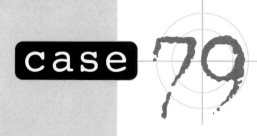

ID/CC A 40-year-old white woman complains of **paleness and bluish discoloration of the hands**, mainly **upon exposure to cold, with redness upon rewarming** (RAYNAUD PHENOMENON); increasing pain in the knees, elbows, and hands over several months; and recent **difficulty swallowing** solid food.

HPI She also has **masklike facies** with a limited range of expression.

PE **Smooth, shiny, tight skin** over face and fingers; edema of hands and feet; palpable subcutaneous **calcinosis; pigmentation** and telangiectasias of face.

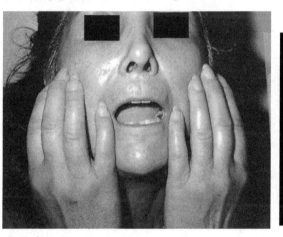

Figure 79-1. Masklike facies and tight skin over fingertips.

Labs CBC: anemia; anti-Scl-70 antibody; positive rheumatoid factor. PFTs: restrictive lung disease (fibrosis).

Imaging UGI: loss of esophageal motility; dilated esophagus.

Gross Pathology Pulmonary fibrosis with "honeycomb" appearance; swelling of esophageal wall; malabsorption syndrome.

Micro Pathology Dense fibrosis of collagen tissue of dermis with loss of appendages and epidermal atrophy; intimal thickening of blood vessels, primarily in kidney.

RHEUMATOLOGY

157

case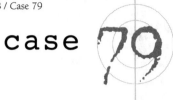

Scleroderma

Differential

Mixed connective tissue disease
Amyloidosis
Carcinoid syndrome
Silicosis
Idiopathic pulmonary fibrosis
Asbestosis

Discussion

Progressive systemic sclerosis (PSS) may be localized or systemic (visceral involvement) and may present with calcinosis, Raynaud phenomenon, esophageal involvement, sclerodactyly, and telangiectasia (CREST SYNDROME).

Treatment

Largely supportive; ACE inhibitors for renal disease; penicillamine or methotrexate for skin thickening; calcium channel blockers or nitrates for Raynaud phenomenon; omeprazole and erythromycin for gastrointestinal dysmotility; cyclophosphamide for pulmonary fibrosis.

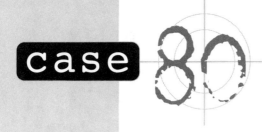

case 80

ID/CC	A 60-year-old woman presents with **swelling and pain** in the left **knee after undergoing a major surgical procedure.**
HPI	She has no history of fever or trauma.
PE	Left knee warm and crepitant upon movement, which is restricted and painful; positive patellar tap indicates an effusion.
Labs	Synovial fluid from left knee shows increased leukocyte count, predominantly neutrophils; normal uric acid levels; **birefringent crystals**, both free and within leukocytes; **calcium pyrophosphate** crystals show a **weakly positive birefringence and are rhomboid in shape.**

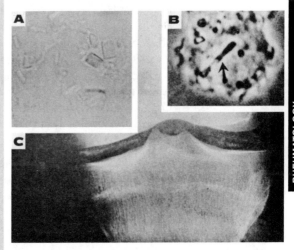

Figure 80-1. Weakly birefringent rhomboid crystals (A); phagocytosed crystals in PMNs (B); linear deposits of crystals in joint space (C).

Imaging	XR, left knee: punctate and **linear calcification in articular cartilage** (CHONDROCALCINOSIS).

RHEUMATOLOGY

case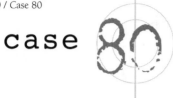

Pseudogout

Differential

Gout

Meniscal tear

Osteoarthritis

Septic arthritis

Spondyloarthropathy

Discussion

The term "pseudogout" refers to acute attacks of arthritis associated with the presence in the synovial fluid of birefringent crystals, both free and within leukocytes. **Pseudogout crystals show a weakly positive birefringence, whereas monosodium urate crystals show a strongly negative birefringence.** Generally, pseudogout crystals are also stubbier and more rhomboid than urate crystals. Radiographic evidence of calcinosis (presumably CPPD crystals) in cartilage and other structures is often present. The typical pattern involves calcification in articular cartilage, fibrocartilage (meniscus of the knee, pubic symphysis, annulus fibrosus), synovium, fibrous capsules, tendons, and bursae. Common sites of involvement include the knee, shoulder, wrist, elbow, hand, and ankle.

Treatment

Anti-inflammatory drugs, including salicylates, phenylbutazone, indomethacin, and glucocorticoids, are effective to varying degrees; joint aspiration may help; triamcinolone intra-articularly for resistant cases.

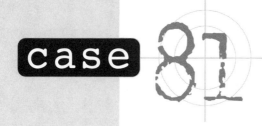

ID/CC A **30-year-old** white **woman** complains that the **fingers** of both hands **become pale** on **exposure to cold.**

HPI At times, the pain is also precipitated by **emotional stress.** She is not taking any drugs and does not suffer from any other diagnosed ailment (e.g., collagen vascular disease; thyroid, adrenal, or pituitary diseases). Symptoms are relieved when she soaks her hands in warm water.

PE Peripheral pulses palpable; **dipping patient's hands in cold water precipitated pain and resulted in development of digital blanching;** rewarming caused cyanosis and rubor of fingers.

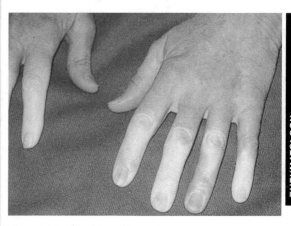

Figure 81-1. Blanching of fingertips.

RHEUMATOLOGY

Labs Pending.

Micro Pathology Arterial wall changes in advanced state of disease.

case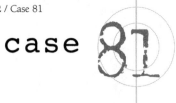

Raynaud Disease

Differential

Frostbite
Cryoglobulinemia
Hepatitis C
Buerger disease
Dermatomyositis
Scleroderma
Rheumatoid arthritis

Discussion

Primary Raynaud phenomenon, or Raynaud disease, is a vasospastic disorder, whereas secondary Raynaud phenomenon occurs as a complication of systemic disease such as scleroderma, systemic lupus erythematosus, and related immunologic disorders. Women are affected approximately five times more than men, and the age at presentation is usually between 30 and 40 years. The fingers are involved more frequently than the toes.

Treatment

Protect hands and feet from exposure to cold; drug therapy with a calcium channel blocker such as nifedipine or a sympatholytic agent such as reserpine or guanethidine; surgical sympathectomy in resistant cases.

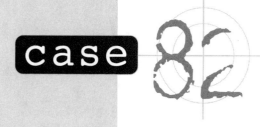

ID/CC   A 23-year-old man presents with bilateral **conjunctivitis**, painful **swelling of the right knee**, bilateral heel pain, and **painless ulcers on his penis**.

HPI   He was diagnosed and treated for nongonococcal urethritis 1 week ago.

PE   Bilateral conjunctivitis with anterior uveitis; **circinate balanitis; kerato-blennorrhagicum on palms and soles;** arthritis of right knee and ankle.

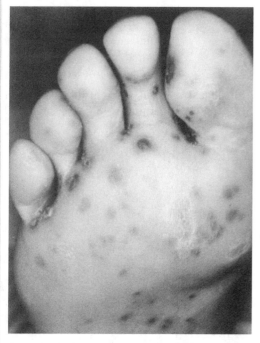

Figure 82-1. Keratoderma blennorrhagicum on the sole.

Labs   **HLA-B27 positive;** synovial fluid reveals monocytes with phagocytosed neutrophils; rheumatoid factor negative; antinuclear antibodies (ANA) negative; elevated ESR.

Imaging   XR, right knee and ankle: presence of **joint effusion**.

163

case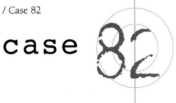

Reiter Syndrome (Reactive Arthritis)

Differential

Ankylosing spondylitis

Gout

Septic arthritis

Rheumatic fever

Psoriatic arthritis

Discussion

Reiter syndrome is an HLA-B27-associated seronegative spondyloarthropathy that is seen almost exclusively in males and is associated with conjunctivitis, urethritis, arthritis, and heel pain. The condition has traditionally been classified as an STD, but it has also occurred following regional enteritis with *Salmonella*, *Shigella*, *Campylobacter*, and *Yersinia*.

Treatment

NSAIDs are mainstay of therapy; treat chlamydial urethritis with doxycycline.

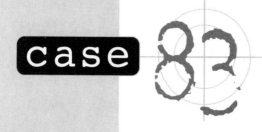
ID/CC   A 47-year-old white **woman** visits her family doctor complaining of painful swelling of the right knee.

HPI   She has **morning stiffness** in the hand joints **lasting** for at least **2 hours**.

PE   **Symmetrical deforming arthropathy** (ulnar deviation); soft-tissue swelling and tenderness in proximal interphalangeal and metacarpophalangeal (MCP) joint; wasting of small muscles of hand; flexion of MCP joint; hyperextension of proximal interphalangeal (PIP) joint and flexion of distal interphalangeal (DIP) joint (SWAN-NECK DEFORMITY).

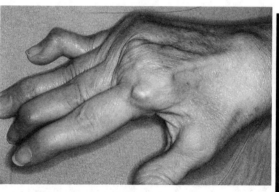

Figure 83-1. Nodule on the metacarpophalangeal joint and swan-neck deformity of the fifth digit.

Labs   Increased ESR; increased protein and white count in the synovial fluid; **positive rheumatoid factor;** positive antinuclear antibodies (ANAs).

Imaging XR, plain: narrowing of joint spaces.

Micro Pathology   Plasma cell infiltration of synovial membranes (SYNOVITIS) with destruction of articular cartilage, tendons, and ligaments by thickened, **inflamed synovial tissue** (PANNUS); **fibrosis.**

RHEUMATOLOGY

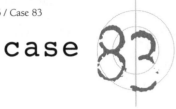

case

Rheumatoid Arthritis

Differential

Carpal tunnel syndrome

Gout

Septic arthritis

Reiter syndrome

Sjögren syndrome

Systemic lupus erythematosis

Discussion

Rheumatoid arthritis is the most **common autoimmune disease.** Ocular involvement is seen in 5% of cases; neurologic involvement of the carpal tunnel can be a complication.

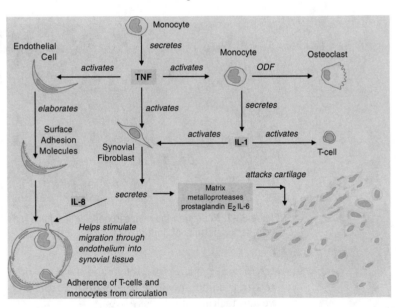

Figure 83-2. Pathogenesis of rheumatoid arthritis.

Treatment

Physical therapy, thermal compresses, splints; NSAIDs; methotrexate; gold; chloroquine; corticosteroids; infliximab or etanercept in selected cases; other immunosuppressants; surgery.

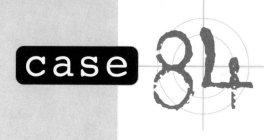

case 84

ID/CC	A 21-year-old college student complains of low-grade fever along with **pain** and **swelling** in her left knee of 5-day duration.
HPI	She had been to her family physician 2 weeks ago because of **dysuria** and a **purulent vaginal discharge** and was given an "antibiotic shot." She was asymptomatic until 4 days ago. She then developed **fever, chills,** and pain in both wrists and in her left ankle, which disappeared when the pain appeared in her left knee (MIGRATORY POLYARTHRALGIA).
PE	**Swollen, tender, warm** left knee with **limited range of motion;** white vaginal discharge. Hemorrhagic skin lesions and pustules on the fingers.

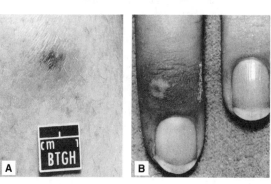

Figure 84-1. Characteristic skin lesions (A); pustulovesicular finger lesions (B).

Labs	**Intracellular, bean-shaped Gram-negative diplococci** and **markedly elevated WBC count** on urethral smear.
Imaging	XR, knee: soft tissue swelling.

case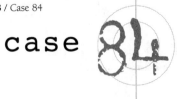

Septic Arthritis—Gonococcal

Differential
Reiter syndrome
Rheumatic fever
Lyme disease
Hepatitis B
Parvovirus infection

Discussion
Almost always accompanied by synovitis and effusion, gonococcal arthritis can rapidly destroy articular cartilage and may be associated with skin rash and C5, C6, C7, and C8 complement deficiencies. Single joints are usually affected, most often the wrists, fingers, knees, and ankles.

Treatment
IV ceftriaxone.

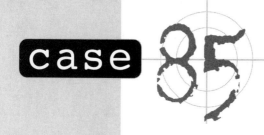

case 85

ID/CC A 47-year-old woman visits her health care center complaining of **dryness of the mouth** (XEROSTOMIA) and a **gritty sensation in her eyes with dryness** (XEROPHTHALMIA).

HPI She has been hypertensive for 20 years and has suffered from long-standing **rheumatoid arthritis**, for which she has been treated with NSAIDs.

PE **Filamentous keratitis with areas of denuded corneal epithelium** (KERATOCONJUNCTIVITIS SICCA) on slit-lamp examination with rose bengal dye staining of cornea; **diminished tear formation** as measured on strip of filter paper, with one end of paper placed inside lower eyelid (SCHIRMER TEST); **parotid enlargement**; excessively dry mouth with abundant dental caries.

Labs Low saliva flow rates with lemon juice stimulation (<0.5 mL/min); hypergammaglobulinemia; **positive antibodies to IgG globulins** (RHEUMATOID FACTOR) and **antinuclear antibodies**; anti-Ro/SSA and anti-La/SSB antibodies positive.

Imaging Sialography (radiography following cannulation and contrast injection of parotid ducts): distortion of normal arborization pattern. Nuc: impaired salivary function.

Micro Pathology Salivary and lacrimal glands show inflammatory infiltration with T cells, B cells, and plasma cells, with predominance of CD4 T cells; **ductal obstruction** with glandular acinar tissue atrophy with fatty change.

RHEUMATOLOGY

case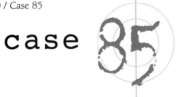

Sjögren Syndrome

Differential | Amyloidosis
Bulimia
Polymyositis
Scleroderma
Pleomorphic adenoma

Discussion | Sjögren syndrome is defined as autoimmune destruction of salivary and lacrimal glands; it may be primary or associated with other autoimmune diseases.

Treatment | Artificial tear preparations, increased and frequent oral intake of fluids, careful dental hygiene, plaque control programs, fluoride application.

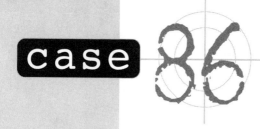
ID/CC	An 18-year-old white **woman** presents with a **malar rash** that is exacerbated by sun exposure (PHOTOSENSITIVITY) as well as with arthralgias and **joint stiffness** involving her ankles, wrists, and knee joints.
HPI	She has a history of hematuria and no history of drug intake prior to the onset of symptoms.
PE	VS: hypertension (BP 160/100). PE: pallor; malar rash; painful restriction of movement of wrist, knee, and ankle joints; no obvious deformity.

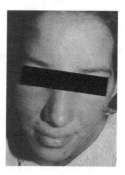

Figure 86-1. Malar rash.

Labs	CBC: Coombs-positive **anemia; neutropenia; thrombocytopenia. Decreased C1q, C2, C4; positive antinuclear antibodies (ANAs), anti-dsDNA, and anti-Sm antibodies**; positive LE cells; false-positive VDRL due to antiphospholipid antibodies. UA: proteinuria; RBCs and **RBC casts.**
Gross Pathology	Serositis; pericarditis; pleuritis; splenomegaly; hyperkeratotic, erythematous plaques.
Micro Pathology	Thickening of basement membrane on renal biopsy; mesangial proliferation; thickened capillary walls, creating **"wire-loop"** appearance, immune complex deposition in skin with lymphocytic infiltration; vasculitis with fibrinoid necrosis of small arteries; almost any organ may be involved.

RHEUMATOLOGY

171

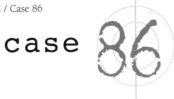

case

Systemic Lupus Erythematosus

Differential | Antiphospholipid syndrome
Fibromyalgia
Infectious mononucleosis
Rheumatic fever
Scleroderma
Lyme disease

Discussion | Systemic lupus erythematosus (SLE) is a **type III hypersensitivity reaction.** Immune complex vasculitis is the basic pathologic lesion; can be drug-induced (e.g., hydralazine, procainamide, isoniazid).

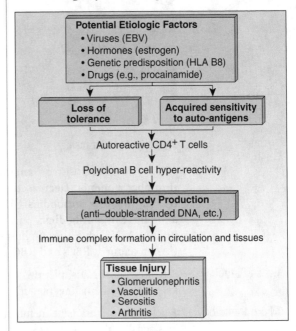

Figure 86-2. Pathogenesis of SLE.

Treatment | High-dose corticosteroids for prolonged periods; alternative drugs: chloroquine; methotrexate; cyclophosphamide as treatment for lupus nephritis.

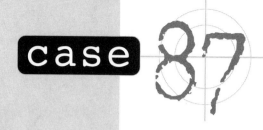

case 87

ID/CC	A 45-year-old **white** man complains of chronic nasal congestion and discharge over the past 5 months.
HPI	Ten days ago he developed an earache and cough along with bloody sputum production, dyspnea, muscle pain, red eyes, fever, and night sweats.
PE	Dried-up crusts of mucus in congestive nasal mucosa with shallow **ulcers and perforation of the nasal septum;** sibilant rales disseminated in lung fields.
Labs	CBC: mild anemia; moderate leukocytosis. UA: numerous RBCs; **red cell casts** and granular casts in urine. **Positive cytoplasmic antineutrophilic antibodies (C-ANCA)** in serum.
Imaging	CXR: bilateral nodular cavitary infiltrates without hilar adenopathy.

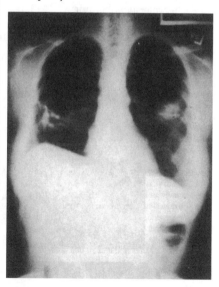

Figure 87-1. Bilateral nodular cavitary infiltrates.

Micro Pathology	Focal necrotizing vasculitis involving small vessels; granulomas and crescentic glomerulonephritis.

RHEUMATOLOGY

173

case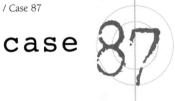

Wegener Granulomatosis

Differential

Glomerulonephritis

Lung abscess

Lung cancer

Pneumonia

Systemic lupus erythematosus

Goodpasture syndrome

Discussion

Wegener granulomatosis is a systemic **autoimmune vasculitis** that consists of necrotizing vasculitis and necrotizing granulomas of the lungs and airways, as well as a necrotizing glomerulitis. C-ANCA is seen in the majority of patients and serves as a marker of disease activity.

Treatment

Immunosuppressive therapy with steroids and cyclophosphamide.

case 88

ID/CC An obese **44-year-old woman** complains of **irritability** and excessive weight gain (40 kg) over the past 3 years and requests medical weight-loss therapy.

HPI On careful questioning, she also reports **easy bruising, oligomenorrhea, weakness, and increased hair growth** in various areas of her body.

PE VS: hypertension (BP 180/110). PE: facial acne; **truncal obesity** with thin extremities; **buffalo hump** and plethoric **moon facies; hirsutism;** wide, purple abdominal and lower leg **striae.**

Labs UA: 3+ **glycosuria. Elevated fasting blood sugar; elevated plasma cortisol;** high ACTH. Lytes: **hypokalemia.** CBC: leukopenia. Low-dose **dexamethasone suppression test** fails to suppress hypercortisolism.

Imaging MR, pituitary: pituitary adenoma. XR, plain: **generalized osteoporosis.** MR, abdomen: bilateral adrenal hyperplasia.

Gross Pathology Pituitary adenoma; bilateral **adrenocortical hyperplasia.**

Micro Pathology Pituitary: benign basophilic adenoma with Crook hyalinization.

case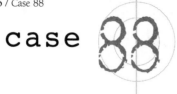

Cushing Syndrome

Differential

Obesity

Hypothyroidism

Exogenous glucocorticoids

Alcoholism

Stress

Discussion

Cushing syndrome comprises the manifestations of hypercortisolism regardless of its cause; causes include excess glucocorticoid administration, paraneoplastic processes (ECTOPIC), ACTH production, adrenal lesions that produce excess cortisol, and pituitary lesions that produce excess ACTH (CUSHING DISEASE).

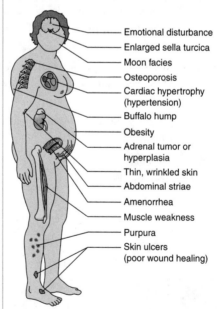

Figure 88-1. Major clinical manifestations of Cushing syndrome.

Treatment

Surgical removal of pituitary adenoma (transsphenoidal adenectomy) or pituitary irradiation along with adjunct medical therapy.

ID/CC   A 40-year-old **woman** is seen in the outpatient clinic with complaints of sudden-onset **painful neck swelling.**

HPI   Prior to this she had a **sore throat, malaise, and fever.** Pain over the thyroid area radiates to the ears and is worse on swallowing.

PE   VS: fever; tachycardia. PE: fine **tremors** of tongue and fingers of outstretched hands; firm, exquisitely **tender, diffuse, mildly enlarged goiter** palpable; nonfirm nodularity felt; no cervical lymphadenopathy; no ophthalmopathy.

Labs   CBC: elevated leukocytes. Elevated ESR; elevated free T_3 and T_4 levels and resin uptake.

Imaging   Nuc: poorly visualized thyroid gland due to markedly **reduced radioactive iodine uptake** (key diagnostic feature and used for differentiating it from Graves disease).

Gross Pathology   Diffusely enlarged thyroid gland; involved areas are firm and yellow against the normal uninvolved brown thyroid substance.

Micro Pathology   Early lesions include **disruption of thyroid follicles with a neutrophilic infiltrate and formation of microabscesses;** subsequently, **multinucleated giant cells** may be seen surrounding colloid fragments, resembling granulomas.

case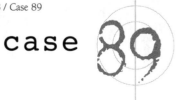

De Quervain Thyroiditis

Differential

Riedel thyroiditis
Radiation thyroiditis
Graves thyrotoxicosis
Toxic multinodular goiter
Thyroid adenoma

Discussion

De Quervain thyroiditis, or subacute **painful** thyroiditis, is the most common cause of severe thyroid pain and tenderness; it is most common in **women 20 to 50 years** of age and shows an association with **HLA-B35.** Its exact etiology is unknown, but viral causes have been implicated.

Treatment

Propranolol and analgesics for symptomatic relief are generally adequate. The condition is **self-limiting,** lasting 6 to 8 weeks. Severe cases may require **prednisone** therapy; permanent hypothyroidism may result on rare occasions, in which case hormone replacement is required. **Antithyroid drugs are not indicated.**

ID/CC   An **8-year-old** black boy is brought to his pediatrician because of a 4-kg **weight loss** over a period of 3 months.

HPI   His mother says that he has also been complaining of **excessive thirst, hunger, and urination** (POLYDIPSIA, POLYPHAGIA, POLYURIA). The patient also reports **waking up several times during the night to urinate** (NOCTURIA).

PE   **Thinly built** male child with an otherwise-normal physical exam.

Labs   **Elevated fasting blood sugar** (180 mg/dL); elevated postprandial blood sugar (270 mg/dL). UA: **glycosuria. Islet cell antibodies** and **anti-insulin antibodies in serum**; elevated glycosylated hemoglobin (hemoglobin A_{1C}).

Micro Pathology   Decreased number of pancreatic β islets with hyalinization, fibrosis, and lymphocytic infiltration.

case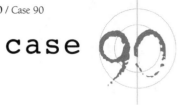

Diabetes Mellitus Type I (Juvenile Onset)

Differential

Diabetes insipidis
Hyperthyroidism
Pheochromocytoma
Steroid treatment
Mature onset diabetes of youth (MODY)

Discussion

Previously known as **insulin-dependent diabetes mellitus** (IDDM), diabetes mellitus type I typically arises before age 20 and is caused by **autoimmune** (T-cell) destruction of β cells. It may be triggered by Coxsackievirus B4, mumps, or other viruses in individuals with a genetic predisposition, and it is linked to **chromosome 6-HLA-DR3 or -DR4.** Close-to-normal values of **glycosylated hemoglobin** reflect good long-term control of blood sugar levels. The main causes of death (in descending order) are myocardial infarction, renal failure, cerebrovascular disease, and infection. Other manifestations include **blindness, retinopathy, peripheral neuropathy,** and **gangrene** of extremities.

Treatment

Glycemic control with insulin therapy; diet and exercise; monitoring hemoglobin A_{1C} levels; prevention, screening, and treatment of comorbid conditions such as hypertension and hyperlipidemia; screening and management of diabetic retinopathy and nephropathy.

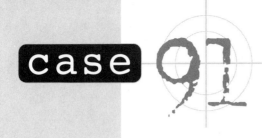

ID/CC An **obese 55-year-old** white man complains of increasing **thirst** and **excessive appetite**.

HPI He also complains of **increased urinary volume**, weight loss, and weakness over the past several months together with burning and **tingling sensations** in a **stocking-glove distribution** (suggesting peripheral neuropathy).

PE VS: hypertension (BP 150/95). PE: **"dot-blot" hemorrhages, exudates, and microaneurysms** on funduscopic exam; muscle atrophy in hips and thighs; diminished dorsalis pedis and tibialis pulses bilaterally.

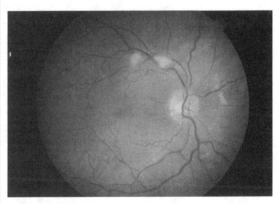

Figure 91-1. "Dot-blot" hemorrhages and exudates seen on funduscopic exam.

Labs **Elevated glycosylated hemoglobin** (HEMOGLOBIN A$_{1c}$). UA: **glycosuria.** Elevated fasting serum glucose (HYPERGLYCEMIA).

Micro Pathology Amyloidosis; hyaline atherosclerosis; nodular hyaline masses (KIMMELSTIEL–WILSON NODULES) in glomerulus.

ENDOCRINOLOGY

case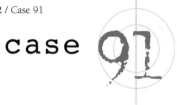

Diabetes Mellitus Type II

Differential

Diabetes mellitus type I
Insulin resistance
Obesity
Stein–Leventhal syndrome

Discussion

Previously known as **non-insulin-dependent diabetes mellitus,** diabetes mellitus type II is a metabolic disease involving carbohydrates and lipids caused by peripheral **resistance to insulin.** Although patients with type II diabetes mellitus are not prone to developing diabetic ketoacidosis, they can develop **nonketotic hyperosmolar coma** if their blood glucose is drastically elevated. Sequelae of type I and type II diabetes mellitus include peripheral vascular disease, coronary artery disease, stroke, diabetic nephropathy, diabetic neuropathy, non-healing skin ulcers, and delayed wound healing with increased risk of infection.

Treatment

Diet and exercise; oral hypoglycemic agents, including sulfonylureas, meglitinides, biguanides, β-glucosidase inhibitors, and glitazones; insulin as needed; screening and management of hypertension and hypercholesterolemia; regular screening and management of diabetic retinopathy and nephropathy.

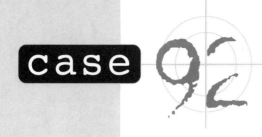

ID/CC A **45-year-old woman** presents with a **swelling in the anterior portion of her neck.**

HPI She also complains of **slowed speech, easy fatigability,** and **cold intolerance.** She is known to have **rheumatoid arthritis,** for which she is taking NSAIDs.

PE **Puffy face; dry skin; coarse hair; swelling of thyroid gland** in anterior portion of neck; swelling is mobile with deglutition but not with protrusion of tongue; thyroid has rubbery consistency; right lobe more enlarged than left; swan neck deformity of left ring finger; ulnar deviation of fingers of both hands.

Labs T_3, T_4 low; TSH high; **antithyroglobulin antibodies** and **antimicrosomal antibodies** (ANTITHYROID PEROXIDASE ANTIBODIES) detected by ELISA.

Imaging Nuc: decreased radioactive iodine uptake (RAIU).

Gross Pathology Diffuse, moderate enlargement of thyroid gland; cut surface is light gray and appears similar to a lymph node.

Micro Pathology Biopsy shows massive infiltration by lymphocytes and plasma cells; normal follicles not present; scant colloid; eosinophilic **Hürthle cell** degeneration seen.

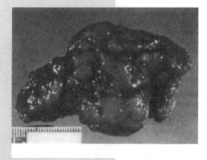 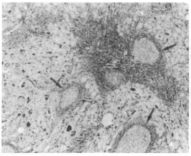

Figure 92-1. Low-magnification photomicrograph showing prominent lymphoid infiltrate with multiple reactive germinal centers *(arrows)*. Many of the follicles are atrophic, and there is scanty colloid.

case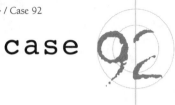

Hashimoto Thyroiditis

Differential

Goiter

Lithium side effect

Hypopituitarism

Polyglandular autoimmune syndrome

Euthyroid sick syndrome

Discussion

Hashimoto thyroiditis is often associated with other autoimmune diseases, including systemic lupus erythematosus, pernicious anemia, Sjögren's syndrome, and chronic hepatitis; it has a genetic association with HLA-DR5 (goitrous form) and HLA-DR3 (atrophic form). Thyrotoxicosis may be seen early in the course of this **autoimmune disease** owing to inflammatory disruption of thyroid follicles (HASHITOXICOSIS).

Treatment

Replacement therapy with **levothyroxine (T$_4$).**

ID/CC   A 24-year-old white woman comes to her family doctor because of **weight loss** despite having a **good appetite**; she also complains of increasing **anxiety**.

HPI   She admits to having frequent bouts of **diarrhea**, reduced sleep capacity, **heat intolerance**, sweaty palms, **palpitations, tremors**, and **menstrual irregularity**.

PE   VS: **tachycardia**. PE: tremors of outstretched hand; **warm, moist skin; right lobe of thyroid palpably enlarged; left lobe not palpable;** no evidence of retrosternal goiter; no cervical lymphadenopathy.

Labs   **Decreased plasma TSH;** increased free T_4 and T_3; antihydroperoxidase antibody absent.

Imaging   Nuc: **hyperfunctioning hot** (increased uptake) thyroid **nodule** with **decreased uptake in surrounding tissue and right lobe** (due to atrophy of remainder of gland secondary to feedback inhibition of TSH).

Gross Pathology   Smooth, rounded, well-circumscribed single mass in right lobe of thyroid gland; no areas of hemorrhage or necrosis; remainder of gland atrophic.

Micro Pathology   No signs of atypia; follicular stroma with abundant, normal-appearing colloid.

case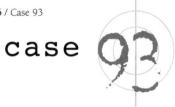

Hyperthyroidism (Solitary Nodule)

Differential

Toxic goiter

Graves disease

Toxic thyroid adenoma

Struma ovarii

Plummer–Vinson syndrome

Discussion

Plummer nodule is a variant of toxic nodular goiter in which hyperthyroidism is caused by overproduction of thyroid hormone by a single thyroid adenoma known as **toxic adenoma.** The most common cause of hyperthyroidism is Graves disease. This autoimmune disease results from antibodies that mimic the TSH molecule, thereby increasing thyroid hormone production.

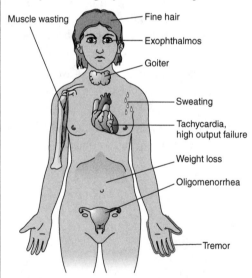

Figure 93-1. Major clinical manifestations of hyperthyroidism (Graves disease).

Treatment

Treat thyrotoxicosis with **propranolol** and antithyroid medications (e.g., propylthiouracil and methimazole); ablation of adenoma by either radioactive iodine or surgery.

case 94

ID/CC	A 46-year-old white man visits his family doctor complaining of **impotence** and **fatigue** over the past year along with **decreased peripheral vision.**
HPI	He also complains of **decreased appetite** and **cold intolerance.** Last week, he scratched both sides of his car while driving through an alley.
PE	VS: **hypotension** (due to decreased ACTH). PE: pallor; **bitemporal hemianopsia** on visual field testing; optic atrophy; loss of axillary and pubic hair; increasingly sparse beard; smooth, dry skin; **testicular atrophy.**
Labs	Lytes: hyponatremia. **Low TSH, ACTH, FSH, and LH;** correspondingly low free T_3, free T_4, cortisol, estrogen, and testosterone; hypoglycemia.
Imaging	CT/MR: **pituitary mass** compressing optic chiasm. XR, skull: widening of sella turcica.
Gross Pathology	Compression of optic chiasm and hypothalamus by pituitary adenoma; may undergo infarction; atrophy of thyroid, testes, and adrenals.
Micro Pathology	Adenoma of chromophobe cells with abundant cytoplasm lacking granules.

case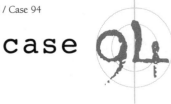

Hypopituitarism

Differential

Kallmann syndrome
Polyglandular syndrome
Empty sella syndrome
Pituitary tumor
Sheehan syndrome

Discussion

The most common cause of hypopituitarism is a pituitary tumor compressing the anterior pituitary. Other common causes are **ischemic necrosis** of the anterior pituitary in postpartum women (SHEEHAN SYNDROME), pituitary surgery/radiation, and, in children, **craniopharyngiomas**.

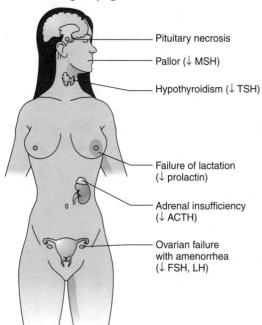

Figure 94-1. Clinical manifestations of panhypopituitarism.

Treatment

Surgical resection (transsphenoidal adenectomy) and hormone replacement (glucocorticoids, levothyroxine [T_4], testosterone).

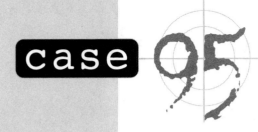

case 95

ID/CC   A 6-year-old boy is brought in for a pediatric consultation due to a hoarse voice, **growth retardation**, and developmental delay.

HPI   The boy's mother describes a **prolonged gestation** and a birth weight of 4.5 kg. The boy has had problems at school owing to a short attention span, sleeping in class, and **mental sluggishness**.

PE   Dry, **yellowish skin**; wide-based ataxic gait; **large tongue** (MACROGLOSSIA); muscular atrophy; **short stature** for age; broad nose; **umbilical hernia**; puffy eyes (due to myxedema) and wide epicanthal distance; slow relaxation of tendon reflexes; thin, brittle hair; **protuberant abdomen**; weak, hoarse voice; goiter.

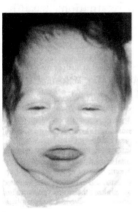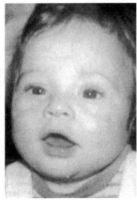

Figure 95-1. Child at 6 months; note myxedema of face, eyelids, lips, and tongue.

Labs   Elevated TSH; low T_3 and T_4.

Imaging   XR, plain: absence of some ossification centers; coxa vara (DECREASED FEMORAL ANGLE); delayed epiphyseal development.

Gross Pathology   Enlarged thyroid gland; **myxedema;** failure of sexual organs to develop properly.

ENDOCRINOLOGY

189

case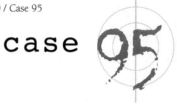

Hypothyroidism—Congenital

Differential

Beckwith–Wiedemann syndrome

Panhypopituitarism

Growth failure

Mental retardation

Hyposomatotropism

Discussion

Congenital hypothyroidism in an infant or child leads to **irreversible mental retardation;** it is caused by lack of iodine, thyroid developmental defects, radioactive iodine exposure during pregnancy, autoimmune disorders, and drugs. Protean manifestations include neuromuscular impairment, short stature (dwarfism), cardiovascular symptoms, and **sexual retardation;** it can be **mistaken for Down syndrome** with grave consequences. All states in the United States currently require neonatal screening for hypothyroidism, galactosemia, and phenylketonuria.

Treatment

Levothyroxine replacement.

ID/CC   A 48-year-old white woman complains of progressive **weakness, lethargy,** and **cold intolerance.**

HPI   She also complains of **weight gain, constipation, coarsening of her facial features,** hair loss, and increasing **hoarseness** in her voice. She adds that her periods have become irregular and heavy. Her husband notes that she has become increasingly forgetful and **depressed.**

PE   VS: bradycardia. PE: coarse facial features; periorbital edema; yellowish skin that is rough, cold, and dry; **brittle, thinning hair; loss of hair of outer third of eyebrows;** cardiomegaly; enlarged tongue; **delayed recovery phase** of Achilles tendon reflex.

Labs   Elevated TSH; low free T_4; elevated serum cholesterol; anti-TPO antibody positive.

Imaging   Nuc: low radioactive iodine uptake (RAIU) by the thyroid.

Micro Pathology   Myxoid degeneration of connective tissue, harboring isolated areas of atrophic follicle; lymphocytic infiltrate seen if Hashimoto thyroiditis is the etiology.

case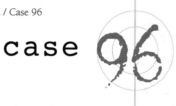

Hypothyroidism—Primary

Differential
Addison disease
De Quervain thyroiditis
Euthyroid sick syndrome
Hypopituitarism
Goiter
Subacute thyroiditis

Discussion
The most common causes of hypothyroidism are **Hashimoto thyroiditis** and hyperthyroidism that has been treated with **surgery** or **radioactive iodine**; it may be **primary** (TSH is high) or **secondary** (low production of TSH by pituitary).

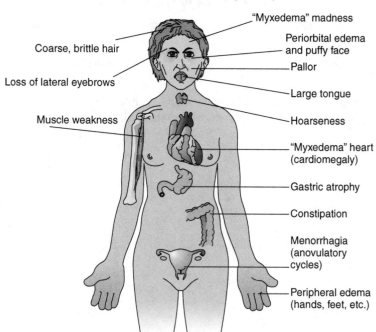

Figure 96-1. Clinical manifestations of hypothyroidism.

Treatment
Levothyroxine (T_4) replacement.

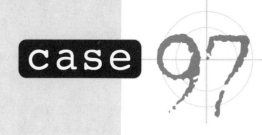
ID/CC	A **7-year-old boy** is brought to a physician for an evaluation of **precocious puberty**.
HPI	He has a history of **severe headaches and visual blurring**.
PE	**Fully developed secondary sexual characteristics** (Tanner stage IV); **paralysis of upward gaze** (PARINAUD SYNDROME); convergence retraction nystagmus; funduscopy reveals **bilateral papilledema**; wide-based gait.
Labs	Elevated CSF β-hCG level.
Imaging	MR, brain (with contrast): **obstructive hydrocephalus and brightly enhancing mass in region of pineal gland**.

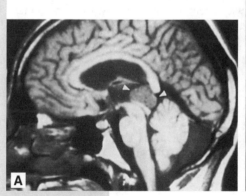
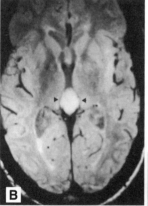

Figure 97-1. Hyperintense mass on T-2-weighted images.

Micro Pathology	Microscopic pathology reveals tumor to be of **germ cell origin**.

case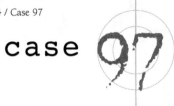

Pinealoma

Differential

Colloid cyst
Craniopharyngioma
Astrocytoma
Meningioma
See below

Discussion

Pineal region tumors include **pineocytomas and pineoblastomas** derived from the pineal parenchymal cells as well as **teratomas and germinomas**; precocious puberty occurs in young males, primarily as a result of **destruction of the pineal gland by a germinoma.** Pinealomas may produce hypothalamic hormone deficiency, leading to hypopituitarism or diabetes insipidus.

Treatment

Because germinomas are extremely radiosensitive, radiotherapy is the mainstay of treatment; often combined with chemotherapy, surgery, shunt placement, and management of endocrinopathies.

ID/CC	A 33-year-old white woman presents with **menstrual cycle irregularity** with long periods of **amenorrhea** and **milky nipple discharge** (GALACTORRHEA).
HPI	Further questioning discloses that she has also **been unable to conceive.**
PE	VS: BP normal. PE: no gynecologic masses palpable; pelvic exam normal.
Labs	**Hyperprolactinemia; reduced LH and estradiol.**
Imaging	MR: enhancing pituitary microadenoma (>10 mm); deviation of pituitary stalk.

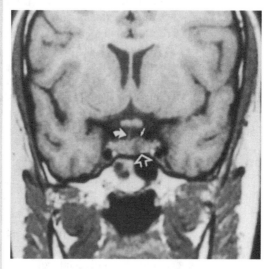

Figure 98-1. Decreased intensity of mass in pituitary (open arrow).

case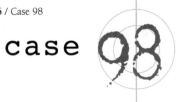

Prolactinoma

Differential

Amenorrhea

Hypothyroidism

Polycystic ovarian syndrome

Antipsychotic medications

Trauma

Discussion

Prolactinoma is the most common type of pituitary adenoma. Hypothalamic GnRH is suppressed by excessive prolactin secretion by the tumor, and thus LH and estradiol are reduced. In **males**, it usually presents as a macroprolactinoma with **headache, impotence,** and **visual disturbance.** Pathologic hyperprolactinemia can also be caused by the interruption of hypothalamic dopaminergic suppression of pituitary prolactin release (e.g., suprasellar masses, pituitary stalk section, and drugs such as haloperidol, phenothiazines, and reserpine). Thus, mild hyperprolactinemia does not always signify the presence of a neoplasm. Elevated estrogen (stimulates lactotrophs) and renal insufficiency are additional causes of hyperprolactinemia.

Treatment

Bromocriptine (dopamine analogue) to inhibit prolactin synthesis and release (and to reduce size of large tumors); consider transsphenoidal surgery in patients whose tumors remain large despite bromocriptine therapy, in those who cannot tolerate dopamine agonists, and in psychiatric patients who require dopamine antagonists.

ID/CC	A 40-year-old woman complains of an unsightly, **progressively increasing neck swelling** and intermittent shortness of breath.
HPI	She has noticed unusually **engorged neck veins** and has recently developed **difficulty swallowing solids** (DYSPHAGIA) and **loud snoring** (STRIDOR) while sleeping. There are **no symptoms of hypothyroidism or hyperthyroidism.** She uses iodized salt (iodine deficiency produces endemic goiter).
PE	PE: anterior, **irregularly surfaced swelling that moves with deglutition** (MULTINODULAR GOITER); percussion over sternum is dull (due to retrosternal extension of goiter); **suffusion of face with marked dyspnea when patient raises both arms** overhead for a few seconds (due to tracheal compression); **no tremors or eye signs**; no cervical adenopathy.
Labs	T_3, T_4 normal; **TSH elevated;** thyroid autoantibodies absent.
Imaging	CXR: **retrosternal extension** of the goiter, producing tracheal compression and deviation. US/CT: **diffuse multinodularity.**
Gross Pathology	Resected **thyroid grossly enlarged;** surface **covered by nodules of varying sizes.**
Micro Pathology	Follicles **distended with colloid;** follicle lining cells flattened; degenerative changes present in between nodules.

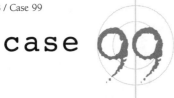

case 99

Sporadic Multinodular Goiter

Differential
Thyrotoxicosis
Thyroid cyst
Thyroiditis
Malignant thyroid tumors
Goiter
Hashimoto thyroiditis

Discussion
The cause of enlargement of the thyroid is most often unknown; known causes include **iodine deficiency** (in endemic areas), **ingestion of goitrogens** (e.g., cabbage, cassava), water pollutants, or **defects** in the synthesis or transport of hormone. In addition to tracheal compression and dysphagia, substernal goiters can also cause phrenic or recurrent laryngeal nerve palsies, esophageal varices, and Horner syndrome.

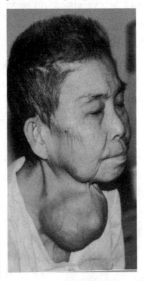

Figure 99-1. Large endemic goiter.

Treatment
Subtotal thyroidectomy for relief of mass effect; **thyroxine** subsequently administered to **suppress** TSH levels and prevent recurrence.

ID/CC A 50-year-old **woman** presents with a **nodule in the front of her neck** that she first noticed 1 month ago.

HPI She notes that the nodule has grown, but she does not complain of any symptoms suggestive of a hyperthyroid or hypothyroid state. She consumes iodized salt. She works as an **x-ray technician** (radiation exposure).

PE **Firm, nontender nodule** in anterior portion of neck, mobile with deglutition; anterior cervical lymphadenopathy; no tremors, sweating, pretibial/pedal myxedema, or exophthalmos.

Labs **Normal thyroid function tests;** normal thyroid hormone levels.

Imaging XR, neck: stippled calcification. Nuc: **cold nodule.** US: **solid nodule.**

Gross Pathology Nodule can range in size from microscopic to several centimeters with invasive margins; may be sclerotic or partly cystic.

Micro Pathology FNA: **psammoma bodies;** lymphocytes; large pink follicular cells with **empty-appearing nuclei** ("Orphan Annie" nuclei) and eosinophilic intranuclear inclusions.

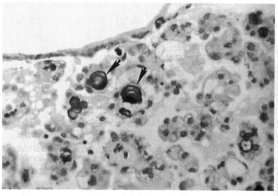

Figure 100-1. Psammoma bodies in the thyroid.

case

Thyroid Carcinoma

Differential

Thyroid lymphoma
De Quervain thyroiditis
Follicular carcinoma of the thyroid
Medullary carcinoma of the thyroid
Anaplastic carcinoma of the thyroid
Papillary carcinoma of the thyroid

Discussion

Ionizing radiation is a predisposing factor for the development of **papillary carcinoma** of the thyroid. Papillary carcinoma spreads via the lymphatics and may present with only cervical lymphadenopathy and an occult primary. In contrast, follicular and sporadic medullary carcinomas commonly metastasize via the bloodstream. Of all histologic variants of thyroid cancer **(papillary, follicular, anaplastic, medullary),** papillary carcinoma carries the best prognosis and anaplastic carcinoma the worst. Medullary carcinoma of the thyroid is derived from **parafollicular cells** (C cells) and is most commonly sporadic, but it may also occur in familial forms with multiple endocrine neoplasia (MEN) types IIA and IIB.

Treatment

Ipsilateral lobectomy and exploration of regional lymph nodes; follow-up levels of serum thyroglobulin; levothyroxine suppression.

questions

1. A 56-year-old man visits his family physician with complaints of "heartburn" despite the use of H2-antagonists. He is markedly overweight and has a 50-pack-year history of smoking as well as drinking a six pack of beer every 2 days. He is referred to a gastroenterologist who performs an esophagogastroduodenoscopy with biopsy. The biopsy demonstrates metaplastic gastric intestinal type columnar epithelial cells. All of the findings suggest the patient likely has which of the following conditions?

   A. Achalasia
   B. Hiatal hernia
   C. Esophageal variceal bleeding
   D. Barrett esophagus
   E. Esophageal carcinoma

2. A 15-year-old boy is brought in by his mother to the family physician. The boy has experienced bouts of abdominal pains along with diarrhea for the last several weeks. He has begun losing weight as he does not experience such symptoms when he does not eat. His uncle has a similar condition for which dietary modification has helped significantly. The doctor suspects celiac disease and, in addition to suggesting a modified diet, sends away lab tests for antibodies. Given the findings, which of the following is likely in this patient?

   A. Anti-endomysial antibodies
   B. Antiparietal cell antibodies
   C. Antimitochondrial antibodies
   D. Anti–smooth muscle antibodies
   E. Antithyroid antibodies

3. A 17-year-old girl is referred to a gastroenterologist with complaints of colicky abdominal pain. She admits to occasional bouts of bloody diarrhea and postprandial bloating. During the last week she has not been able to eat much and admits to a 5-lb weight loss over the last month. Her mother has a history of inflammatory bowel disease for which she has had a partial bowel resection. A colonoscopy is performed and there are areas of discontinuous inflammation. Biopsy results return with a diagnosis of Crohn disease. Which of the following was likely seen on biopsy?

A. Mallory bodies
B. Transmural inflammatory changes
C. Mucosal and submucosal herniations through the muscular layer
D. Crypt abscesses
E. Flattening and atrophy of the mucosal villi

4. A 45-year-old man presents to his family physician for a yearly physical. The patient notes that over the last year people have asked him if he has been "tanning" as his skin appears bronze. As well, they have noted a "yellow hue" to his eyes. On exam he does have scleral icterus and a palpably enlarged liver. Labs return with a serum glucose of 250 g/dL. A diagnosis of hemochromatosis is suggested. What is the best screening test for this condition?

A. Serum ferritin levels
B. Serum bilirubin levels
C. Antibodies to *Saccharomyces cerevisiae*
D. Serum ammonia levels
E. Genetic testing for HFE mutations

5. A 30-year-old recent immigrant from Ghana presents to a county hospital with complaints of abdominal distension. He also complains of a 20-lb weight loss over the last months. On exam, the patient has a noticeable temporal wasting and a palpably enlarged liver. A CT scan of the abdomen detects a large solitary liver mass. Labs demonstrate an elevated α-fetoprotein but an elevated carcinoembryonic antigen. Exposure to which of the following would likely contribute to the patient's state?

A. Hepatitis A
B. Asbestos
C. Human papillomavirus
D. Aflaxotoxin B
E. Aniline dyes

6. A 15-year-old girl complaining of abdominal pain is taken to the physician for an evaluation. Her mother had similar complaints several years ago and had a colonoscopy performed. At that time, biopsy demonstrated multiple heavy and pedunculated growths of the jejunum, ileum, and colon. The patient has obvious hyperpigmented macules on her lips and buccal mucosa; however, no other physical exam findings. The likely diagnosis in this case is:

A. Hereditary nonpolyposis colon cancer syndrome
B. Gardner syndrome
C. Osler–Weber–Rendu syndrome
D. Familial polyposis syndrome
E. Peutz–Jeghers syndrome

7. A 24-year-old man has visited the gastroenterologist on numerous occasions with complaints of burning epigastric pain. Initially, he was given H2 blockers with no relief. At that point the EGD was performed demonstrating erosive growth without evidence of *Helicobacter pylori*. He was given a proton pump inhibitor, again without relief. The gastroenterologist orders a fasting serum gastrin, which returns dramatically elevated. Which of the following is the likely diagnosis?

A. WDHA syndrome
B. Carcinoid syndrome
C. Whipple triad
D. Zollinger–Ellison syndrome
E. Meckel diverticulum

8. A 57-year-old man is brought to the emergency room by his wife. For several days, he experienced wild flailing movements of his left arm and leg only. On exam, there are no nonfocal neurologic symptoms other than the chief complaint. His other medical conditions include uncontrolled diabetes and hypertension. He has no other remarkable family history of any conditions. Which of the following will likely be found in this patient?

A. Bilateral temporal lobe and amygdala damage
B. An infarct in the dominant inferior frontal gyrus
C. Degeneration and atrophy of the neurons of the corticospinal tracts and anterior motor neurons of the spinal cord
D. Atrophy of the caudate nucleus
E. An infarct in the contralateral subthalmic nuclei

9. A 12-year-old girl is brought to the pediatrician with complaints of a severe headache and vomiting. She also complains of vision changes and frequent urination. She is noticeably shorter than children her age. On exam, she demonstrates papilledema and a CT scan is ordered. The scan demonstrated a suprasellar mass with ring calcifications. A transsphenoidal biopsy is performed and the pathology report comments on the "remnants of Rathke pouch" being noted. Which of the following is most likely?

A. Medulloblastoma
B. Craniopharyngioma
C. Pseudotumor cerebri
D. Neuroblastoma
E. Pituitary adenoma

10. A 60-year-old man complains of an extreme headache and nausea that is worse in the morning. At work, he experiences a seizure and is brought to the emergency room by ambulance. A CT scan of the head is performed and it demonstrates an enhancing mass with a necrotic center and adjacent edema. A high-grade astrocytoma is suspected, and he is taken for a total gross resection by neurosurgery. Final pathology returns which of the following?

A. Pseudopallisading of tumor cells
B. Antoni A and Antoni B histologic patterns
C. "Fried egg" appearance of tumor cells
D. Psammoma bodies
E. Perivascular pseudorosettes

11. A 45-year-old school teacher complains of bilateral lower extremity weakness. She notes the weakness has been progressively moving up on her legs. Two weeks earlier, she recalls suffering from a bout of bloody diarrhea and fever. Soon after admission, she experiences respiratory distress requiring intubation. A diagnosis of Guillain–Barré syndrome is suspected. Which of the following is consistent with this diagnosis?

A. Spongiform change within the cerebral cortex
B. Gross distension of the endolymphatic system
C. Marked loss of cells in the posterior root ganglion and degeneration of peripheral sensory fibers
D. Multiple ring enhancing lesions at the gray/white junctions of the cerebrum
E. Increased CSF protein concentration without cellular increase

12. A 19-year-old woman complains of generalized weakness. She is seen by her family physician who notes significant left-sided ptosis and comments on the development of an increasingly nasal voice of the patient as the interview continues. She is ultimately referred to a neurologist who administers endrophanium in the office with dramatic reversal of the patient's ptosis and weakness. Given these findings a diagnosis of myasthenia gravis is made. Further workup ensues. It would not be uncommon to find which of the following?

A. Berry aneurysm
B. Dermatitis herpatiformis
C. Sclerosing cholangitis
D. Lambert–Eaton myasthenic syndrome
E. Thymoma

13. A 63-year-old man is brought to the family physician by his caretaker, his grandson. The grandson has noted deterioration of the patient's cognitive skills. The patient has also developed bowel and bladder incontinence. He is referred to a neurologist who performs a lumbar puncture to find a normal opening pressure and normal levels of glucose, cells, and protein. A CT scan demonstrates ventricular enlargement with little cortical atrophy. Which is the likely diagnosis?

A. Alzheimer disease
B. Normal pressure hydrocephalus
C. Myotonic dystrophy
D. Internuclear ophthalmoplegia
E. Pseudobulbar palsy

14. A 50-year-old woman presents to the emergency room with a headache and blurred vision for several weeks. She has a few healing bruises on her arms and legs, which she attributes to a minor accident she had when she hit her head on the windshield of her car. At that time, she felt fine and did not seek medical attention, since she had no insurance, and only hit a tree. A CT scan of her head demonstrates a crescenteric accumulation of blood along the skull. Which of the following is most likely?

A. Subarachnoid hemorrhage
B. Capsular infarct
C. Subdural hematoma
D. Hypertensive cerebral accident
E. Epidural hematoma

15. A 16-year-old boy is seen by his family physician with complaints of progressive back pain and stiffness. He notes the pain is worse during the diving session, as he is a varsity athlete on the team. The patient has marked tenderness over the sacroiliac joints. A plain film of the spine demonstrates fusion of the vertebrae in the lumbar area that appears as a "bamboo spine." This inflammatory condition is associated with which of the following autoimmune markers?

A. HLA–DR3 or HLA–DR4
B. HLA B-27
C. Rheumatoid factor
D. HLA–B35
E. Antimicrosomal antibodies

16. A 35-year-old woman complains of discoloration of her hands when she goes out into the cold without gloves. She notes that they return to their normal color when they become warm. She also complains of increasing joint pain as well as palpable swollen joints. Labs are ordered for a complete rheumatologic workup. Given the clinical picture, which is most specific for this patient's presentation?

A. Anti-Sm antibodies
B. Anti-RNP antibodies
C. Autoantibodies to tRNA
D. Anti-Ro and Anti-La antibodies
E. Anti-Scl-70 antibodies

17. A 50-year-old man presents with crampy abdominal pain, fever, and a livedo reticuloris rash on his lower extremities. He also presents with complaints of joint pain. He is given a prompt referral to a rheumatologist. Labs are ordered for a workup demonstrating the patient to have an elevated ESR, p-ANCA antibodies, a positive HbsAg, but no c-ANCA antibodies. What is the likely diagnosis?

A. Pseudogout
B. Wagener granulomatosis
C. Polyarteritis nodosa
D. Polymyalgia rheumatica
E. Syringomyelin

18. A 34-year-old woman presents to the family physician with complaints of painless swelling in her neck. She is hyperviligent, since she had been treated with radiation and chemotherapy for a lymphoma. On exam, she has a palpable nodule on the left hemithyroid. She is referred to a surgeon who performs a core needle biopsy. The diagnosis of papillary carcinoma of the thyroid is made. Which of the following histologic findings was likely present?

A. Tumor cells surrounded by an amyloid stroma
B. Massive infiltrates of the lymphocytes with germinal center formation
C. Undifferentiated cells with frequent mitosis and nuclear atypia
D. Multinucleated giant cells and granuloma formation
E. "Orphan Annie" nuclei in cells

19. A 14-year-old boy has an acute viral illness from which he recovers. Within a week of the resolution of his infection he begins feeling thirsty all the time and begins to eat constantly without gaining weight. He notes not feeling too well and his mother takes him to the emergency room where his blood sugar is reported to be 450 mg/dL (normal 100 mg/dL). After further evaluation he is diagnosed with diabetes mellitus. What is the most likely mode of inheritance?

   A. X-linked dominant
   B. Autosomal dominant
   C. Autosomal recessive
   D. Multifactorial
   E. Mitochondrial

20. Your 42-year-old patient presents as she begins to develop bizarre involuntary spasmodic twitching or jerking movements and noticed her memory has been getting progressively worse. She notes that her mother developed similar symptoms at the age of 62 and was subsequently diagnosed with Huntington disease. She was hoping she would not manifest with the symptoms until she was a similar age and wondered why she was beginning to be affected so early. This can be, in part, a result of what genetic phenomena?

   A. Lyonization
   B. Anticipation
   C. Imprinting
   D. Inversion
   E. Aneuploidy

answers

1-D

  A. Achalasia [Incorrect] This results from a loss of ganglion cells in the myenteric plexus of the esophagus, which could be apparent in a biopsy. Patients with this condition present with difficulty swallowing liquids and solids.

  B. A hiatal hernia [Incorrect] This results from a weakness in the diaphragm with protrusion of the stomach through the diaphragmatic crura. Although a hiatal hernia may predispose to the development of Barrett esophagus, not everyone with a hiatal hernia will develop Barrett esophagus, and vice versa.

  C. Esophageal variceal bleeding [Incorrect] Patients with portal hypertension may have dilated submucosal veins and varices. On occasion, esophageal variceal bleeding can occur and may be life threatening.

  D. Barrett esophagus [Correct] Patients with long-standing gastrointestinal reflux disease can develop Barrett esophagus. Exposure to stomach GERD could result in metaplasia of the epithelial cells, which further predisposes to cancer.

  E. Esophageal carcinoma [Incorrect] This often presents as an ulcerative mass in the lumen. Untreated Barrett esophagus can result in the development of this cancer, which has a poor prognosis.

2-A

  A. Anti-endomysial antibodies [Correct] Patients with celiac disease have a hypersensitivity to the protein gladin (gluten) found in wheat. Patients experience immune-mediated damage to enterocytes when gluten is not restricted from their diet. Diagnosis is often confirmed by anti-endomysial antibodies and/or antigliadin antibodies.

  B. Antiparietal cell antibodies [Incorrect] These result in loss of parietal cells of the stomach and therefore loss of HCl production as well as decreased intrinsic factor production. Patients develop atrophic gastritis and pernicious anemia.

  C. Antimitochondrial antibodies [Incorrect] Primary biliary cirrhosis is a chronic progressive liver disorder that occurs predominately in middle age. It ultimately develops into potentially fatal liver failure and is associated with the presence of antimitochondrial antibodies.

D. Anti–smooth muscle antibodies [Incorrect] Autoimmune hepatitis is clinically indistinguishable from chronic viral hepatitis. However, it is diagnosed with elevated levels of anti–smooth muscle antibodies.

E. Antithyroid antibodies [Incorrect] Patients with Hashimoto thyroiditis, the most common cause of hypothyroidism, experience autoimmune destruction of the thyroid. Diagnosis is confirmed with the presence of antithyroid antibodies.

3-B

A. Mallory bodies [Incorrect] Patients with alcoholic liver disease demonstrate hepatocellular necrosis and neutrophilic infiltrate on liver biopsy. They also have characteristic eosinophilic hyaline inclusions, known as Mallory bodies.

B. Transmural inflammatory changes [Correct] Crohn disease is an inflammatory bowel disease that is characterized by discontinuous involvement of the bowel (skip lesions), particularly the terminal ileum. However, the lesions do involve the entire depth of the bowel, and so transmural inflammatory changes are visible on biopsy.

C. Mucosal and submucosal herniations through the muscular layer [Incorrect] Diverticulosis, a common condition in older patients, results from the herniation of the mucosa and submucosa through weaknesses in the muscularis layer. Sometimes, these areas become infected, leading to diverticulitis.

D. Crypt abscesses [Incorrect] These are localized areas of inflammatory cell infiltration into the crypts of Lieberkuhn. These lesions are characteristic of ulcerative colitis and inflammatory bowel disease with continuous involvement of the mucosa of the colon.

E. Mucosal villi [Incorrect] The inflammatory infiltrate of the small intestine in patients with celiac sprue results in destruction of the absorptive enterocytes. As such, the brush border is not well developed and there is flattening and atrophy of the mucosal villi.

4-A

A. Serum ferritin levels [Correct] Patients with hemachromatosis, known as bronze diabetes, have a triad of cirrhosis, diabetes mellitus, and skin pigmentation. The disease is caused by an overload of iron, which deposits in several organs, including the heart, pancreas, liver, and skin. Patients have dramatically elevated serum ferritin, and this is the preferred screening test.

B. Serum bilirubin levels [Incorrect] Serum bilirubin is a relatively nonspecific marker of liver disease as well as hemolysis.

C. Antibodies to *Saccharomyces cerevisiae* [Incorrect] Patients with Crohn disease often have antibodies to *Saccharomyces cerevisiae*. Although not a screening test, such findings might be helpful in differentiating Crohn disease from ulcerative colitis, and therefore guide therapy in patients with inflammatory bowel disease.

D. Serum ammonia levels [Incorrect] A principal function of the liver is to clear serum ammonia from the blood. In patients with severe liver disease, ammonia accumulates causing encephalopathy.

E. Genetic testing for HFE mutations [Incorrect] Although patients with hemochromatosis have genetic mutations in a protein involved in iron metabolism, HFE, genetic testing is not the recommended screening test for the diagnosis of the disorder. Once patients are found to have an increased ferritin, it may be appropriate to consider genetic testing for such mutations.

5-D

A. Hepatitis A [Incorrect] Although hepatitis B (HBV) and hepatitis C (HCV) are closely associated with the development of hepatocellular carcinoma, hepatitis A (HAV) is a self-limiting condition without sequelae.

B. Asbestos [Incorrect] Exposure to asbestos is a significant risk factor for the development of mesothelioma, a malignant tumor of the pleural lining. The risk is even greater with concurrent tobacco use. However, there is no association with liver cancer.

C. Human papillomavirus (HPV) [Incorrect] Cervical cancer is a leading cancer among women worldwide, and human papillomavirus (HPV) is a major contributor to this cancer. HPV also is associated with tumors of the head and neck.

D. Aflatoxin B1 [Correct] This is a carcinogen produced by molds on grains. It is a common problem in developing nations, as they attempt to deal with the nutritional needs of their populations. As well, it synergizes with HBV in the development of hepatocellular carcinoma.

E. Aniline dyes [Incorrect] Like those used in the textile industry, aniline dyes are carcinogens implicated in the development of the transitional cell carcinoma of the urinary tract.

6-C

A. Hereditary nonpolyposis colon cancer syndrome [Incorrect] Patients with this condition have a strong family history for the development of colon cancer. The disorder results from a defect in DNA repair.

B. Gardner syndrome [Incorrect] This is an autosomal dominant condition, characterized by the presence of numerous adenomatous polyps, as well as the presence of soft tissue tumors.

C. Osler–Weber–Rendu syndrome [Correct] Although there are no polypoid lesions identified, patients with Osler–Weber–Rendu syndrome do have telangectasias of the gastrointestinal tract, which are prone to bleed on occasion. This is a hereditary condition that is found more commonly in the Mormon population in Utah.

D. Familial polyposis syndrome [Incorrect] This is an autosomal dominant condition, due to mutations on chromosome 5. The disorder is characterized by the development of thousands of adenomatous polyps of the colon with the aggregate increase in the chance of malignant transformation. Such patients have a nearly 100% chance of developing colon cancer by the fourth decade.

E. Peutz–Jeghers syndrome [Incorrect] This is an autosomal dominant condition, characterized by the development of multiple pigmentary lesions on the mucous membranes, as well as multiple benign colon polyps.

7-D

A. WDHA syndrome [Incorrect] This is seen in patients with tumors that overproduce vasoactive intestinal proteins (VIP). Patients with VIPoma have watery diarrhea, hypocalemia, and achlorydia (WDHA syndrome).

B. Carcinoid syndrome [Incorrect] Overproduction of a metabolite of serotonin, 5-hydroxy indole amino acid (5-HIAA) occurs in patients with carcinoid syndrome. Such patients present with flushing, diarrhea, and endocarditis.

C. Whipple triad [Incorrect] Insulinomas, due to tumors of the beta cells of the pancreas, cause severe hypoglycemia. Patients with such tumors present with Whipple triad. episodic hypoglycemia, CNS dysfunction, dramatically reversed by glucose administration.

D. Zollinger–Ellison syndrome [Correct] Hypersecretion of gastrin is associated with Zollinger–Ellison syndrome. Such patients have recurrent gastric ulcers, refractory to medical management. Gastrinomas are often malignant.

E. Meckel diverticulum [Incorrect] This is a congenital malformation found in 2% of the population. This remnant of the embryonic vitalline duct may have ectopic gastric, duodenal, or colonic tissue.

8-E

A. Bilateral temporal lobe and amygdala damage [Incorrect] Patients with Kluver–Bucy syndrome manifest with hyperphagia, hypersexuality, and hyperorality. Such patients have damage to their bilateral temporal lobes and amygdala.

B. An infarct in the dominant inferior frontal gyrus [Incorrect] Broca area is located in the dominant inferior frontal gyrus. Therefore, patients with an infarct in this region experience an expressive aphasia—known as Broca aphasia.

C. Degeneration and atrophy of the neurons of the lateral corticospinal tract and anterior motor neurons of the spinal cord [Incorrect] These result in amyotrophic lateral sclerosis (ALS) or Lou Gehrig disease. ALS is a progressive neurologic disease, ultimately resulting in death due to complications of respiratory paralysis.

D. Atrophy of the caudate nucleus [Incorrect] This is found in patients with Huntington disease. These patients also experience jerky movements of their extremities; however, this is typically bilateral.

E. An infarct in the contralateral subthalmic nucleus [Correct] The patient in this vignette presents with the classic symptoms of hemiballismus. This condition, due to an infarct in the contralateral subthalmic nucleus, results in loss of control of the extremities of the opposite side of the body.

9-B

A. Medulloblastoma [Incorrect] This is one of the most common intracranial neoplasms in children. However, it is often a malignant tumor of the cerebellum, located in the posterior fossa.

B. Craniopharyngioma [Correct] The pituitary gland is derived embryologically from the Rathke pouch. Craniopharyngiomas are tumors of the sella, derived from this embryonic tissue. Symptoms are due to hypopituitarism (growth retardation and diabetes insipidus), as well as mass effects (bilateral hemionapsia, headache, and vomiting).

C. Pseudotumor cerebri [Incorrect] This can indeed cause headaches and increased intracranial pressure. It most commonly occurs in overweight females.

D. Neuroblastoma [Incorrect] Tumors of the sympathetic ganglia and adrenal are referred to as neuroblastomas. The most common location of this tumor is the adrenal medulla. These tumors are associated with the overexpression of the N-myc oncogene.

E. Pituitary adenoma [Incorrect] Although pituitary adenomas can present with symptoms of mass effects, they often present with symptoms due to overproduction of pituitary hormones (hyperprolactinemia). As well, craniopharyngiomas are the most common suprasellar tumors in children.

10-A

A. Pseudopallisading of tumor cells [Correct] This patient likely has the highest grade astrocytoma, a glioblastoma multiforme, based on the presence of necrosis. Histologically, these tumors have areas of necrosis and hemorrhage, surrounded by "pseudopalisade" arrangement of tumor cells.

B. Antoni A and Antoni B histologic patterns [Incorrect] Histologically, schwannomas (tumors arising from Schwann cells) are characterized by two distinct histologic patterns: Antoni A and Antoni B. The Antoni A pattern is characterized by interlacing bundles of elongated cells and the Antoni B pattern is looser, less cellular.

C. "Fried-egg" appearance [Incorrect] Oligodendrogliomas are characterized by closely packed cells with large round nuclei surrounded by a clear halo of cytoplasm. This results in a characteristic "fried egg" appearance.

D. Psammoma bodies [Incorrect] Meningiomas, benign tumors of the meninges, are characterized by the presence of laminated calcifications, known as psammoma bodies.

E. Perivascular pseudorosettes [Incorrect] Medulloblastomas, the most common intracranial neoplasm in children, are characterized by perivascular pseudorosettes.

11-E

A. Spongiform change within the cerebral cortex [Incorrect] Creutzfeldt–Jakob disease is due to a proteinaceous infectious agent (prion) and can be transmitted by transplanted cornea and dura matter grafts as well as contaminated surgical instruments. The disease causes loss of neurons with spongiform change within the cerebral cortex.

B. Gross distention of the endolymphatic system [Incorrect] This can be seen in patients with Meniere disease. These patients present with recurrent attacks of vertigo, hearing loss, and tinnitus.

C. Marked loss of cells in the posterior root ganglion and degeneration of peripheral sensory fibers [Incorrect] Friedreich ataxia is an autosomal dominant condition resulting in gait disturbance and degeneration of peripheral sensory fibers.

D. Multiple ring enhancing lesions of the gray/white junctions of the cerebrum [Incorrect] These are characteristic of brain metastasis. Tumors of the lung and breast frequently metastasize to the brain.

E. Increased CSF protein concentration without cellular increase [Correct] Patients with Guillain–Barré syndrome experience progressive ascending motor weakness that is often transient and reversible. It is believed to be an autoimmune phenomenon related to viral or bacterial infections. Patients have characteristic CSF findings, demonstrating increased CSF protein without an increased cellularity, a concept known as albuminocytologic dissociation.

12-E

A. Berry aneurysm [Incorrect] Rupture of a berry aneurysm is the most common cause of a subarachnoid hemorrhage. This congenital weakness in the vessels of the circle of Willis is associated with polycystic kidney disease.

B. Dermatitis herpatiformis [Incorrect] Patients with a celiac disease often have an associated skin condition, known as dermatitis herpatiformis. This condition is characterized by pruritic blistering of the extensor surfaces of the body.

C. Sclerosing cholangitis [Incorrect] This is marked by inflammation, fibrosis, and stenosis of hepatic bile ducts. It is closely associated with ulcerative colitis.

D. Lambert–Eaton myasthenic syndrome [Incorrect] This is a paraneoplastic syndrome that develops in patients with small cell carcinoma of the lung. The disorder is characterized by antibodies to presynaptic calcium channels and presents similarly to myasthenia gravis.

E. Thymoma [Correct] This occurs in 20% of patients with myasthenia gravis. Diagnostic workup includes ruling out the presence of this benign tumor of the thymic epithelium.

13-B

A. Alzheimer disease [Incorrect] This is one the most common forms of senile dementia. However, it is generally not associated with bowel or bladder incontinence and will likely demonstrate cortical atrophy on imaging of the head.

B. Normal pressure hydrocephalus [Correct] It is important to recognize the findings of gait disturbance, dementia, and bladder incontinence as a clinical picture associated with normal pressure hydrocephalus (NPH). This form of dementia is potentially reversible with the placement of a ventriculoperitoneal shunt.

C. Myotonic dystrophy [Incorrect] This is a progressive muscular disorder due to an autosomal dominant mutation in the myotonin protein kinase gene. Patients develop distal muscle weakness, facial muscle weakness, frontal balding, and atrophic testicles.

D. Internuclear ophthalmoplegia [Incorrect] The findings of one eye that does not adduct with the other eye with nystagmus on abduction suggests internuclear ophthalmoplegia (INO). This condition is often found in patients with multiple sclerosis.

E. Pseudobulbar palsy [Incorrect] This can result from motor neuron diseases, multiple sclerosis, or bilateral cerebral vascular accidents of the internal capsule. Patients present with difficulty swallowing, nasal regurgitation of food, and spastic weakness of the lower extremities.

14-C

A. Subarachnoid hemorrhage [Incorrect] This typically presents with acute headaches, often described as "worst headache of my life." On CT scan, hyperdense blood can be seen in the cisterns and sulci.

B. Capsular infarcts [Incorrect] These often cause hemiparesis of the contralateral limbs. Often, these result from thrombotic phenomena as in atrial fibrillation.

C. Subdural hematoma [Correct] Laceration of the bridging veins between the dura and arachnoid is often associated with head trauma. This is often a slow accumulation of blood, given the lower pressure of the venous system. Symptoms of a subdural hematoma take weeks to evolve.

D. Hypertensive cerebral vascular accident [Incorrect] Patients with uncontrolled blood pressure are at risk for the development of hypertensive cerebral vascular accident. Often there is rupture of small penetrating arterioles of the putamen, thalamus, pons, and cerebellum.

E. Epidural hematomas [Incorrect] Skull fractures are commonly associated with the rupture of the middle minengeal artery. Such bleeds result in epidural hematomas, which are more rapidly life-threatening. They appear as lens-shaped convexities on head imaging.

15-B

A. HLA-DR3 or HLA-DR4 [Incorrect] Autoimmune diabetes, diabetes mellitus type I, results from autoimmune destruction of the insulin-producing beta cells of the pancreas. The T-cell destruction of beta cells is closely linked to patients who have the HLA class two alleles, HLA-DR3 or HLA-DR4.

B. HLA-B27 [Correct] Ankylosing spondylitis is an autoimmune condition that affects the spines of young men. This condition, along with the rheumatologic conditions, including reactive arthritis (formerly known as Reiter syndrome) and inflammatory bowel disease are associated with the haplotype HLA-B27.

C. Rheumatoid factor [Incorrect] This is an IgM antibody directed to the Fc portion of the IgG antibody. It is present in patients with rheumatoid arthritis as well as other rheumatologic conditions, however, not in patients with ankylosing spondylitis.

D. HLA-B35 [Incorrect] De Quervain thyroditis is a painful inflammatory condition of the thyroid. Although poorly understood, it is thought to result from a viral infection in women, most commonly in those with the haplotype HLA-B35.

E. Antimicrosomal antibodies [Incorrect] These are directed against thyroid peroxidase. They are found in patients with Hashimoto thyroditis.

16-E

A. Anti-Sm antibodies [Incorrect] Patients with systemic lupus erythematosus (SLE) present with joint stiffness, constitutional symptoms, and a characteristic malar rash. Diagnosis of SLE is associated with anti-Sm antibodies as well as anti-dsDNA.

B. Antiribonuclear protein (RNP) antibodies [Incorrect] These are found in patients with mixed connective tissue disease. This disorder presents with a constellation of findings of many rheumatic conditions, including rash, dysphagia, arthralgia, muscle weakness, and Raynaud phenomena.

C. Autoantibodies to tRNA [Incorrect] Dermatomyositis is a rheumatologic condition associated with a heliotopic rash. It can be seen as a paraneoplastic syndrome in patients with lung or ovarian cancer. Patients have antibodies to various tRNAs.

D. Anti-Ro and Anti-La antibodies [Incorrect] Sjögren syndrome is an autoimmune condition affecting primarily middle-aged women. They present with dry mouth (xerostomia), dry eyes (xeropthalmia), and arthritis. Diagnosis is aided by the presence of anti-Ro and anti-La antibodies.

E. Anti-Scl-70 antibodies [Correct] This patient has classic findings of scleroderma, a variant condition known as CREST syndrome (calcinosis, Raynaud phenomena, esophageal involvement, sclerodactyly, telangiectasias). These patients have antibodies to anti-Slc70.

17-C

    A. Pseudogout [Incorrect] Pseudogout results from the accumulation of calcium pyrophosphate dehydrate crystals in articular spaces. The crystals are weakly positively birefringent.

    B. Wegener granulomatosis [Incorrect] Patients with Wegener granulomatosis have cytoplasmic antineutrophilic antibodies (C-ANCA) in their serum. The condition manifests with upper respiratory symptoms with necrotizing granulomas, as well as vasculitis in the lungs and kidneys.

    C. Polyarteritis nodosa [Correct] This is a type III hypersensitivity reaction with involvement of the kidneys, heart, lung, and retina. It is marked as one of the only arteritis that is more common in males. Patients have P-ANCA antibodies and often there is an association with HBV infection.

    D. Polymyalgia rheumatica [Incorrect] This involves stiffness of the muscles of the shoulder and hip girdles. These patients have dramatically elevated ESRs, but no other diagnostic markers. There is significant overlap in patients with temporal arteritis.

    E. Syringomyelin [Incorrect] Patients with Syringomyelin have progressive anesthesia and weakness of both arms, as well as occipital headaches and a shifting gait. This disorder results from central cavitation of the spinal cord.

18-E

    A. Tumor cells surrounded by an amyloid stroma [Incorrect] Medullary carcinoma of the thyroid is a tumor if the C cells of the thyroid. These cells are often surrounded in the amyloid stroma composed of calcitonin.

    B. Massive infiltrates of the lymphocytes with germinal center formation [Incorrect] The most common cause of hypothyroidism is Hashimoto thyroiditis. This condition is histologically characterized by massive infiltrates of lymphocytes with germinal center formation.

    C. Undifferentiated cells with frequent mitosis and nuclear atypia [Incorrect] Of all the types of carcinoma of the thyroid, anaplastic carcinoma has the worst prognosis. This tumor is characterized by undifferentiated cells with frequent mitosis and nuclear atypia.

    D. Multinucleated giant cells and granuloma formation [Incorrect] De Quervain thyroiditis is a painful condition that presents with neck swelling. Biopsy of the thyroid in these patients would demonstrate multinucleated giant cells and granuloma formation.

E. "Orphan Annie" nuclei in cells [Correct] Papillary carcinoma of the thyroid is closely associated with radiation exposure. The prognosis is very good in patients; however, when metastasis occurs it does so via the bloodstream. Pathology reveals large follicular cells with empty-appearing nuclei, so-called "Orphan Annie nuclei."

19-D

A. X-linked dominant [Incorrect] Diabetes mellitus is not an example of a disorder resulting from X-linked dominant mutations. An example of such a disorder such is fragile X syndrome.

B. Autosomal dominant [Incorrect] These mutations usually occur in proteins that form structural proteins or multimeric enzymes. This is because of the concept of "poisoned partners" or the "one bad apple spoils the lot" in which it only takes one aberrant subunit to cause dysfunction in the multimeric unit.

C. Autosomal recessive [Incorrect] There are rare cases in which diabetes can be inherited as a single gene mutation that is inherited in an autosomal recessive fashion, as is the case of maturity onset diabetes of the young (MODY), although these comprise a small fraction of all those with diabetes.

D. Multifactorial [Correct] Diabetes mellitus is an example of a multifactorial disorder, which likely involves multiple genes as well as environmental influences.

E. Mitochondrial [Incorrect] Mitochondrial transmitted defects refer to a small group of defects in genes found in the mitochondrial genome, and are thus maternally inherited, and typically involve oxidative phosporlyation enzymes.

20-B

A. Lyonization [Incorrect] This refers to random inactivation of the X chromosome; this occurs in the cells of females randomly. The product of this inactivated chromosome is a Barr body.

B. Anticipation [Correct] This occurs with trinucleotide repeat disorders with expansion of the repeats from generation to generation, often leading to earlier and more severe symptoms of the disease.

C. Imprinting [Incorrect] This implies that both maternal and paternal sequences are not always equivalent. Some genes need to be inherited equally from each parent; when this does not occur, diseases like Angelman syndrome or Prader–Willi syndrome can occur.

D. Inversions [Incorrect] These result from chromosomal breakage and rejoining during meiosis.

E. Aneuploidy [Incorrect] This results when there is an abnormal number of chromosomes, i.e., a number that is not a multiple of 23. This occurs in the various trisomies or in Turner syndrome.

credits

Austen KF, Frank MM, et al. *Samter's Immunologic Diseases,* 6th Ed. Philadelphia: Lippincott Williams & Wilkins, 2001. Figs. 45.3 (Case 87), 49.1 (Case 92).

Bear MF, Connors BW, Parasido MA. *Neuroscience—Exploring the Brain,* 2nd Ed. Philadelphia: Lippincott Williams & Wilkins, 2001. (Case 35).

Becker KL, Bilezikian JP, Brenner WJ, et al. *Principles and Practice of Endocrinology and Metabolism,* 3rd Ed. Philadelphia: Lippincott Williams & Wilkins, 2001. Figs. 7.8A (Case 39), 47-4 (Case 95), 40-3 (Case 100).

Bhushan V, Le T, Pall V. *Underground Clinical Vignettes: Step 1 Pathophysiology II,* 4th Ed. Malden, Mass: Blackwell Publishing, 2005. Figs. 022 (Case 22), 042 (Case 45), 059 (Case 62), 062 (Case 65), 064 (Case 67).

Bickley LS, Szilagyi P. Bates' *Guide to Physical Examination and History Taking,* 8th Ed. Philadelphia: Lippincott Williams & Wilkins, 2003. (Case 35).

Eisenberg RL. *Clinical Imaging: An Atlas of Differential Diagnosis,* 4th Ed. Philadelphia: Lippincott Williams & Wilkins. Figs. GI 1-4A (Case 1), GI 53-1 (Case 8), GI 1-6 (Case 13), C 25-3 (Case 15), B 33-19 B (Case 36), SK 30-2 B (Case 38), SK 3-1 (Case 54), SK 4-3 (Case 61-1), SP 23-2 (Case 66), SK 24-17 (Case 68), SK 9-5 (Case 97), SK 8-1 (Case 98).

Goodheart HP. *Goodheart's Photoguide of Common Skin Disorders,* 2nd Ed. Philadelphia: Lippincott Williams & Wilkins, 2003. Fig. 25.24 (Case 86).

Greenberg MJ, Hendrickson RG. *Greenberg's Text-Atlas of Emergency Medicine.* Philadelphia: Lippincott, Williams & Wilkins, 2004. Figs. 23-15 A & B (Case 69), 23-17 (Case 79), 23-18 (Case 81).

Humes HD. *Kelley's essentials of internal medicine,* 2nd ed. Philadelphia: Lippincott Williams & Wilkins; 2001:T76-4. (Case 73)

Koopman WJ, Moreland LW. *Arthritis and Allied Conditions: A Textbook of Rheumatology,* 15th Ed. Philadelphia: Lippincott Williams & Wilkins, 2004. Figs. 85.3 (Case 67), 75.1 A & B (Case 71), 61.1 (Case 72), 75.3 A (Case 78), 116.1 (Case 80), 64.4 A (Case 82), 45.12 (Case 83), 52.2 (Case 83), 125.1 A & B (Case 84).

Lawrence PF. *Essentials of general surgery,* 4th ed. Philadelphia: Lippincott Williams & Wilkins; 2006:T18-3. (Case 23)

Mullholland MW, Lillemoe KD, Doherty GM, et al. *Greenfield's Surgery: Scientific Principles & Practice,* 4th Ed. Philadelphia: Lippincott Williams & Wilkins, 2005. Fig. 51-3 (Case 10).

Pilliteri A. *Maternal and Child Nursing,* 4th Ed. Philadelphia: Lippincott Williams & Wilkins, 2003. (Case 91).

Rowland LP. *Merritt's Neurology,* 11th Ed. Philadelphia: Lippincott Williams & Wilkins, 2005. Figs. 34.1 (Case 40), 36.8 (Case 42), 64.8 (Case 43), 64.7 (Case 43), 106.2 (Case 46), 39.1 (Case 47), 60.8A (Case 51), 121.1 (Case 57), 126.4 (Case 58), 49.6 (Case 60).

Rubin E, Farber JL. *Pathology,* 3rd Ed. Philadelphia: Lippincott Williams & Wilkins, 1999. Figs. 13-6B (Case 3), 14-46A (Case 4), 5-7 (Case 8), 21-41 B (Case 59).

Rubin E, Gorstein F, Schwarting R, et al. *Rubin's Pathology: A Clinicopathologic Approach.* 4th Ed. Baltimore: Lippincott Williams & Wilkins, 2004. Figs. 13-60 (Case 9), 14-45 (Case 16), 14-17 (Case 17), 13-9 (Case 25), 13-49 (Case 30), 8-10 (Case 33), 28-58 (Case 38), 28-72 (Case 41), 28-120 (Case 48), 28-99 (Case 50), 28-130 (Case 51), 25-48 (Case 52), 28-141 (Case 53), 26-14 C (Case 74), 26-29 (Case 75), 4-25 (Case 86), 21-36 (Case 88), 21-16 (Case 93), 21-4 (Case 94), 21-12 (Case 96), 21-11A (Case 99), T6-4 (Case 44).

Schiff ER, Sorrell MF, Maddrey WC. *Schiff's diseases of the liver,* 9th ed. Philadelphia: Lippincott Williams & Wilkins; 2003:T53-1. (Case 19)

Swischik LE. *Emergency Imaging of the Acutely Ill or Injured Child,* 4th Ed. Philadelphia: Lippincott, Williams & Wilkins, 2000. Fig. 8.23 A (Case 29).

Tasman W, Jaeger E. The Wills Eye *Hospital Atlas of Clinical Ophthalmology,* 2nd Ed. Philadelphia: Lippincott Williams & Wilkins, 2001. Fig. 9.15 (Case 56).

Yamada T, Alpers DH, et al. *Textbook of Gastroenterology,* 4th Ed. Philadelphia: Lippincott Williams & Wilkins, 2003. Figs. 61-1C (Case 5), 142-35A (Case 6), 138-21 (Case 7), 89-2 (Case 9), 87-2 (Case 11), 33-3 (Case 14), 116-2 (Case 18), 90-5 (Case 24), 143-17 (Case 26), 155-12 (Case 27), 75-3 (Case 31).

case list

GASTROINTESTINAL

1. Achalasia
2. Ascending Cholangitis
3. Barrett Esophagus
4. Budd–Chiari Syndrome
5. Candida Esophagitis
6. Celiac Disease
7. Chronic Atrophic Gastritis
8. Chronic Pancreatitis
9. Colonic Polyps
10. Crohn Disease
11. Diverticulitis
12. Diverticulosis
13. Esophageal Spasm
14. Esophageal Variceal Bleeding
15. Gastroesophageal Reflux Disease
16. Hereditary Hemochromatosis
17. Hepatic Cirrhosis
18. Hepatic Encephalopathy
19. Hepatitis—Alcoholic
20. Hepatocellular Carcinoma
21. Hepatorenal Syndrome
22. Metastatic Carcinoma—Liver
23. Pancreatitis—Acute
24. Peutz–Jeghers Syndrome
25. Plummer–Vinson Syndrome
26. Primary Biliary Cirrhosis
27. Protocolitis
28. Traveler's Diarrhea
29. Toxic Megacolon
30. Ulcerative Colitis
31. Whipple Disease
32. Zollinger–Ellison Syndrome

NEUROLOGY

33. Alcoholism
34. Amyotrophic Lateral Sclerosis
35. Aphasia—Broca Area
36. C1 Spinal Cord Injury
37. Cauda Equina Syndrome
38. Cerebral Aneurysm
39. Craniopharyngioma
40. Creutzfeldt–Jakob Disease
41. CVA, Capsular Infarct
42. CVA, Hypertensive
43. Epidural Hematoma
44. Friedreich Ataxia
45. Glioblastoma Multiforme
46. Guillain–Barré Syndrome
47. Hemiballismus
48. Huntington Chorea
49. Internuclear Ophthalmoplegia
50. Klüver–Bucy Syndrome
51. Medulloblastoma
52. Ménière Disease
53. Meningioma
54. Metastatic Brain Tumor
55. Migraine
56. Multiple Sclerosis
57. Myasthenia Gravis
58. Myotonic Dystrophy
59. Neuroblastoma
60. Normal Pressure Hydrocephalus
61. Oligodendroglioma
62. Peripheral Neuropathy—Diabetic
63. Pseudobulbar Palsy
64. Subarachnoid Hemorrhage

65. Subdural Hematoma
66. Syringomyelia

RHEUMATOLOGY
67. Temporal Arteritis
68. Von Hippel–Lindau Disease
69. Ankylosing Spondylitis
70. Decompression Sickness
71. Dermatomyositis
72. Juvenile Rheumatoid Arthritis
73. Mixed Connective Tissue Disease
74. Osteopetrosis
75. Osteoporosis
76. Polyarteritis Nodosa
77. Polymyalgia Rheumatica
78. Polymyositis
79. Scleroderma
80. Pseudogout
81. Raynaud Disease
82. Reiter Syndrome (Reactive Arthritis)

83. Rheumatoid Arthritis
84. Septic Arthritis—Gonococcal
85. Sjögren Syndrome
86. Systemic Lupus Erythematosus
87. Wegener Granulomatosis

ENDOCRINOLOGY
88. Cushing Syndrome
89. De Quervain Thyroiditis
90. Diabetes Mellitus Type I (Juvenile Onset)
91. Diabetes Mellitus Type II
92. Hashimoto Thyroiditis
93. Hyperthyroidism (Solitary Nodule)
94. Hypopituitarism
95. Hypothyroidism—Congenital
96. Hypothyroidism—Primary
97. Pinealoma
98. Prolactinoma
99. Sporadic Multinodular Goiter
100. Thyroid Carcinoma

index